The New Healers

ALSO BY WILLIAM R. CLARK

The Experimental Foundations of Modern Immunology

*At War Within: The Double-Edged Sword of
the Immune System*

Sex and the Origins of Death

The New Healers

The Promise and Problems of
Molecular Medicine in the
Twenty-First Century

William R. Clark

New York   Oxford
OXFORD UNIVERSITY PRESS
1997

Oxford University Press

Oxford   New York
Athens   Auckland   Bangkok   Bogotá   Bombay
Buenos Aires   Calcutta   Cape Town   Dar es Salaam   Delhi
Florence   Hong Kong   Istanbul   Karachi
Kuala Lumpur   Madras   Madrid   Melbourne
Mexico City   Nairobi   Paris   Singapore
Taipei   Tokyo   Toronto   Warsaw

and associated companies in
Berlin   Ibadan

Copyright © 1997 by Oxford University Press

Published by Oxford University Press, Inc.
198 Madison Avenue, New York, New York 10016

Oxford is a registered trademark of Oxford University Press

Library of Congress Cataloging-in-Publication Data
Clark, William R., 1938–
The new healers : the promise and problems of molecular
medicine in the twenty-first century / by William R. Clark.
p. cm.
Includes bibliographical references and index.
ISBN 0-19-511730-1 (cloth)
1. Gene Therapy—Popular works. I. Title.
RB155.8.C53 1997
616'.042—DC21   97-9086

9 8 7 6 5 4 3 2 1

Printed in the United States of America
on acid-free paper

Contents

Prologue

We watched him on television as he played inside his plastic bubble. We and the rest of the world marvelled that a tiny toddler who had never felt his mother's skin, or smelled her body, or tasted hot food could grow into a bright-eyed, mischievous, highly intelligent and seemingly well-adjusted youth. And then he died. And we mourned, and we asked why.

Young David — the "Bubble-boy," as he came to be known — had SCID: severe combined immune-deficiency disease. SCID is one of an estimated 4,000 human diseases caused by a defective gene, a tiny snippet of one of the forty-six long strands of DNA stored in each of our cells. Children born with SCID have a defect in their immune systems; they are born the immunological equivalent of an AIDS patient entering the final stage of disease, and have about the same life expectancy. They usually die of the same causes — mortal infection by microbial pathogens.

Infectious diseases were once the scourge of the human race, felling the majority of people before they even reached reproductive age. That changed with improved public health programs in major population centers, immunization with crippled forms of microbial pathogens that induce immune protection without causing disease, and finally with the discovery of antibiotics. Before the AIDS epidemic, it was rare (although certainly not unknown) for someone to die of an infectious disease in industrialized countries.

But when all of the diseases caused directly by microbial pathogens are accounted for, human beings still find themselves assaulted by a wide range of crippling, even lethal maladies. These are diseases that are *idiopathic*, arising within us because of some defect in the myriad molecules involved in the construction and operation of the enormously complex human body. A significant portion of these diseases are genetic in origin. Human beings have on the order of 100,000 different genes, instructions written into our DNA for production of the proteins we use to organize and direct every aspect of our biological existence. Defects in the genes encoding any one these proteins can lead to disastrous consequences for the individual inheriting them. The resulting genetic diseases, including such familiar disorders as muscular dystrophy, cystic fibrosis, and sickle cell anemia, can be every bit as devastating as infectious disease, and in one way they are much worse: we pass them on to our children, generation after generation after generation.

Having survived the onslaught of microbial pathogens, we now find ourselves prey to an estimated 4,000 of these genetically based diseases. Science and medicine have provided us with clues to the treatment of some of them, but by the very nature of these diseases they have never been considered curable. The best that could be imagined is that, knowing the particular protein lacking as a result of a deficient gene, we might be able to administer that protein as a form of medicine. Unfortunately, in all but a very few cases it is simply not possible to deliver the missing protein where it is needed, when it is needed.

All of that is about to change, and it is going to change through one of the most profound revolutions in modern medicine, *gene therapy*, a branch of the brand new field of *molecular medicine*. Advances in the laboratory over the past two decades are about to be brought into the clinic; in fact they are already arriving. Progress in the newest field of biology, molecular biology, has made it possible to isolate human genes, to make billions of copies of them in the laboratory, and to reintroduce them into those unfortunate individuals who have inherited damaged or functionless genes. This same technology turned around on itself can be used to introduce deliberately "bad" genes to attack and destroy unwanted cells, such as cancer cells or cells infected with the AIDS virus.

Molecular medicine, particularly in the form of gene therapy, will be a major part of our lives in the new millenium. The success rate of gene therapy at present is modest at best; the number of patients who have been unambiguously cured by it can probably be counted on the fingers of one hand. But the logic behind molecular medicine is powerful and compelling. Everything we know about molecular biology tells us it can work, and that it will work. The federal government and private industry are both betting on it, to the tune of tens of billions of dollars. Over one hundred clinical trials based on this new science are already underway.

Not only doctors, but politicians, attorneys, ethicists, and common citizens will find themselves in the position of having to make personal and professional decisions based on a technology that has taken molecular biologists the better part of half a century to develop. Within the next ten years we will have used that technology to "read" all 100,000 or so genes that make up the human genome. That is easily the medical equivalent of going to the moon; it will take human beings to a completely new level of understanding of our biological selves. We must begin now to think about how we will manage that understanding, and how we will use the information we gain.

Many of us are still recovering from the shock of having computers forced into our lives. But just as computers have changed our lives forever, so too will the tools of molecular medicine, and we will simply have to do what we did with computers: learn to understand them well enough to take advantage of the incredible benefits they can bring us. To do so, we will not all have to earn Ph.D.'s in molecular biology, any more than we had to become mathematicians or electrical engineers to learn how to use computers. The basic elements of molecular biology necessary to understand molecular medicine are easily within the grasp of anyone willing to devote a few hours of thought and reflection. This book will serve as an introduction to this important new frontier of human medicine, and can act as a bridge to the future—a future as exciting and as full of promise as anything we have witnessed in the past century of remarkable progress.

The New Healers

1

In the Beginning

The Discovery of Genes

The story of molecular medicine begins with the story of genes. It is not at all an understatement to say that life as we know it could not exist without genes. They direct the activity of every living organism, from the simplest single-cell bacteria to human beings. Genes are found in and are responsible for the day-to-day operation of every single cell in our bodies; they help us to respond to changes in the environment by directing individual cells to alter the amounts and types of molecules they synthesize. Genes are also the basic units of heredity, and as such are responsible for the transmission of biological characteristics from one generation to the next.

Genes have been around for as long as life has been present on earth, yet their very existence was unknown until the latter part of the last century, and our understanding of them is still evolving. They were first defined in connection with their role in heredity; their parallel role in directing cellular activity was not understood until well into the twentieth century. Beginning with the ancient Greeks, there had been a vague notion that something physical—contributed by both a male and a female in the case of animals, including humans—is involved in heredity, and that this physical substance is able in some fashion to direct the creation of a new being sharing many characteristics of the parents. But it was also recognized that often neither the appearance nor the behavior of an offspring could be predicted in detail from a close study of the parents. During the nineteenth century, for reasons we shall discuss shortly, interest in the biological and ultimately the chemical basis of heredity intensified considerably. Many hypotheses to explain inheritance were put forward, based on things such as the "mixing of blood," or the blending of "forces" or "essences"; none of these ideas compelled serious belief among more than a handful of people. Until very recent times, as John Moore has pointed out in his book, *Science As a Way of Knowing*, fairly sophisticated scientific thinkers did not really even know what questions to pose about biological inheritance.

The possibility of manipulating the inheritance of biological traits, such as size or the ability to resist certain diseases, had long been noted by farmers and used for the selective breeding of animals and plants with desirable characteristics. This practical experience confirmed the correlation of heredity with reproduction, and contributed the important general notion that individual properties of a plant or animal can be manipulated without changing the organism's overall characteristics. The very fact that the inheritance of separate characteristics can be manipulated independently of one another also supports the idea that inheritance is based on physically discrete entities. These entities are what ultimately came to be known as genes.

Gregor Mendel and the Discovery of Genes

The first experiments to provide direct evidence for the existence of genes as we now think of them were carried out in the middle of the last century by Gregor Mendel, an Augustinian monk with a lifelong interest in biology but relatively little formal biological training. Born Johann Mendel in the Silesian region of the Austrian empire in 1822 (the same year in which Louis Pasteur was born), he took monastic vows and the name Gregor at the Königskloster at Altbrünn (now in the Czech Republic) in 1843. He became a priest there in 1847, and abbot in 1868. During these years Mendel carried out a long, intensive study in the monastery garden on inheritance in the common pea plant, *Pisum sativum.*

Mendel focused on the transmission from generation to generation of such physical properties as plant size, seed shape and color, flower shape and color, and pod color. Mendel's basic approach was to generate hybrids by cross-fertilizing strains of plants that bred true for different characteristics. After eight years of work, he presented his results publicly in two 1865 lectures, which were published the following year under the title *Versuche über Pflanzen-Hybriden* (*Experiments with Plant Hybrids.*)

Prior to Mendel, most scientists thought that when plants or animals with slightly different characteristics were bred, the offspring tended to be more or less intermediate in their biological properties between the two parents. At the level of an entire individual, this may seem to be true. Mendel's great contribution was to show through careful analysis that when single, specific traits of an individual are followed in an isolated fashion from one generation to the next, this turns out not at all to be true. For example, when pea plants producing only smooth peas were bred to plants producing only wrinkled peas, the hybrid offspring did not produce "slightly wrinkled" or "mostly smooth" peas; they produced only perfectly smooth peas, just like the smooth-pea parent. The smooth characteristic is completely dominant over wrinkled. But Mendel showed clearly that the *potential* to make a wrinkled pea is still present in the hybrid. If the hybrid plants are bred among themselves, approximately one-quarter of *their* progeny will be wrinkled, even though all of the hybrid parents themselves produced only smooth peas.

Where did the wrinkled peas go in the hybrid plants? What happened to them? How did they resurface in the next generation? The ability of an organism to pass on to its offspring traits that the organism does not itself express was not entirely unknown; people often talk about characteristics that "skip a generation." But it was Mendel's determination to understand the underlying basis for this phenomenon that led to one of his most important contributions to modern biology. By carrying out large numbers of experiments and carefully tabulating the results, Mendel realized that not only were these "invisible" traits preserved and passed on to the next generation, but they were *always passed on in a specific and reproducible ratio* (Figure 1-1). Mendel's great contribution was to recognize that when natural phenomena occur in a mathematically predictable fashion, they must have a rational and mathematically expressible basis. It

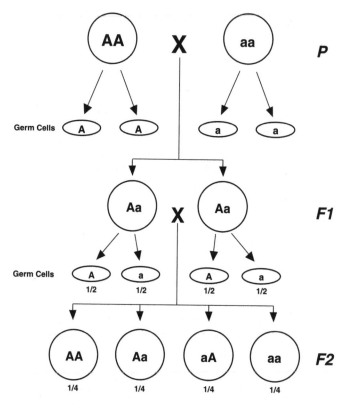

Figure 1-1. Basic Mendelian genetics.

was his dogged insistence on this point that seems to have put off his contemporaries but which ultimately secured his place in the history of science.

Mendel argued that his observations could only be explained by postulating the existence of multiple, independent hereditary "elements" or "units," essentially proposing the existence of what we now call genes. He concluded that each of the characteristics of the pea plant that he was studying must be controlled by a separate heredity element. For each given element (let us use the word "gene" from now on, even though Mendel himself did not*), Mendel postulated there would be multiple

---

*The word "gene" was first suggested only in 1909, by the Danish biologist Wilhelm Johannsen, to define the elements that control heredity. By that time scientists were fully convinced of the correctness of Mendel's ideas, and were fairly sure that the substance of heredity was associated with material stored in the nucleus of each cell in the body.

forms present in the population. For example, Mendel proposed that the gene controlling pea shape must exist in at least two forms: one that can cause peas to be wrinkled, and one that causes peas to be smooth. These alternate forms of the same gene are now called *alleles*. Mendel showed very clearly that the ratios of transmission he observed could only be explained if each organism inherits two alleles (one from each parent) for each different gene. Importantly, Mendel also showed that the maternally inherited and paternally inherited alleles do not fuse or combine or blend in any way; they remain separate, intact, and integral throughout the life of the individual inheriting them, and can be passed on separately and individually to the next generation. Thus each adult organism has two alleles of each gene, but passes on only one of these alleles (randomly selected) to each offspring. The genes are passed forward in special cells called *germ cells*, which we will discuss shortly.

In order to explain the apparent disappearance of a given trait in one generation, only to reappear in the next, Mendel introduced the concept that some alleles are dominant over others—smooth over wrinkled, for example. If the alleles for smooth and wrinkled are present in the same pea plant, the peas produced by that plant will all be smooth, because smooth is dominant. That is how some alleles can seem to be invisible in a given generation. A plant that has both "wrinkled" and "smooth" alleles, and thus produces only smooth peas, will nonetheless be able to pass the "wrinkled" allele on to its offspring, a portion of which will produce wrinkled peas. However, in order to produce wrinkled peas, plants must inherit only the "wrinkled" allele from both parents; Mendel termed such alleles recessive. The condition of having two identical alleles of the same gene (whether dominant or recessive) is known as *homozygosity*; having a mixture of two different alleles is known as *heterozygosity*. Only plants homozygous for the recessive "wrinkled" gene will produce wrinkled peas. Plants homozygous for "smooth" or heterozygous for "smooth/wrinkled" will both produce only smooth peas, leading to the 3:1 ratio of smooth:wrinkled offspring in the F2 generation in Figure 1-1. (This brings up the important concepts of *genotype* vs. *phenotype*. Genotype is the precise combination of alleles of different genes possessed by a given individual, for example Aa in Figure 1-1. Phenotype is basically what the organism looks like as the result of the genotype. The phenotype of both AA and Aa in Figure 1-1 is smooth, even though the genotypes are different.)

Mendel's second major contribution was to demonstrate scientifically what farmers had known intuitively all along: genes controlling one characteristic, such as pea shape, can function completely independently of genes controlling other properties such as flower shape or pod color. Most importantly, these genes can behave independently during reproduction. For example, consider two distinct genes in pea plants: the one that controls, in different allelic forms, wrinkled vs. smooth seeds (peas), and another gene whose alleles are responsible for the color of the seed pods, green or yellow. For the latter gene, green is dominant over yellow. As shown in Figure 1-2, a plant heterozygous for both of these genes can transmit to its offspring either the dominant or the recessive allele for each gene. But the choice of allele transmitted in each case is random, independent of and unaffected by the choice of allele in the other case. As a result, the germ cells of such a plant will each contain one of four different genotypes. If mated with another plant heterozygous for both of these genes, sixteen different kinds of offspring can be produced in terms of genotype, but only four distinct phenotypes result. (An important restriction on this phenomenon of independent gene *segregation*, caused by the physical association of genes with individual chromosomes, will be discussed below.)

Mendel's Impact on Biology. Mendel is often depicted as working in intellectual isolation, a monk who was struck by a biological epiphany that allowed him to create completely new ideas in an arena where nothing had existed before. It does not at all detract from Mendel's great contributions to realize that his work was in fact a logical extension of the plant breeding experiments carried out by a number of scientists before him, most notably Josef Kölreuter at the end of the 18th century, and Carl von Gärtner beginning in the 1820s. Kölreuter developed the notion that plants, like animals, engage in sexual reproduction and are subject to similar laws of heredity. He developed most of the techniques of cross-fertilization and hybridization that would underlie Mendel's experiments, and defined the role of wind and insects in distributing pollen, which would be crucial to Mendel in controlling his own experiments. Von Gärtner, whose work was extensively read and quoted by Mendel, also worked with peas and described qualitatively many of the same phenomena reported by Mendel. Mendel acknowledged his predecessors fully in his famous paper.

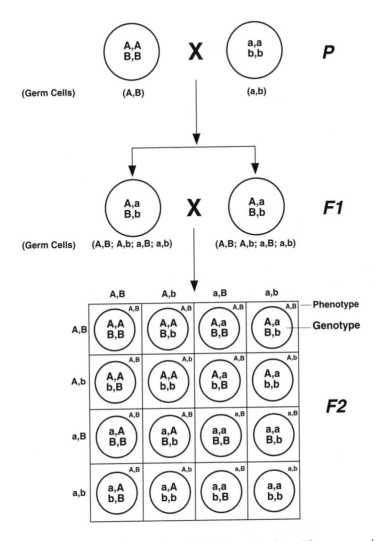

Figure 1-2. Genes can segregate independently during breeding. The upper case letters represent the dominant allele of each gene; the lower case letters are the recessive alleles. Notice what happens in the F2 generation: both the dominant and the recessive alleles from one parent segregate independently, pairing with either a dominant or recessive allele from the other parent at either gene. The result is sixteen different genotypes, with four distinct phenotypes: A,B (9/16); A,b (3/16); a,B (3/16); a,b (1/16).

But only Mendel, sorting through column upon column of what must have seemed to many at the time mind-numbing statistics, understood the implications of the precise and reproducible ratios of traits segregating into offspring. Only Mendel saw that just as complex physical materials such as sand or rocks or metals can be understood on the basis of the properties of the individual atoms from which they are made, so too can a complex living organism be understood as the sum of its biological and hereditary "atoms"—its genes. Mendel's insights into heredity have often been compared with those of Dmitri Ivanovich Mendeleyev, the Russian chemist whose understanding of the underlying mathematical relationships among atoms led to his formulation of the periodic law of chemical elements, which underlies all modern chemistry. In fact, what little formal scientific training Mendel had was actually in physics, with its underlying mathematics.* This doubtless prepared him to think about his breeding observations in ways very different from his predecessors and peers in plant breeding, and perhaps explains their inability to appreciate what he was trying to convey.

Unfortunately, Mendel was unable to propose for his genes either a physical form or an anatomical association. Nor did he formulate his ideas into a working hypothesis that could be understood in relation to what was then known about biology, or that suggested further experimentation. Thus his "elements" remained simply abstract algebraic symbols to be moved around on paper in order to explain inheritance. To those few biologists who read his paper, if they managed to plow through his statistics, it was not immediately obvious that Mendel's hypothesis about heredity was any more valid than anyone else's. That realization would come only when other scientists carried out the same kind of extensive and detailed breeding programs as Mendel did, and subjected them to the same kind of rigorous mathematical analysis, but in the context of specific chemical and biological structures. That would not happen for another thirty years.

From statements he made in his original paper, it seems likely that Mendel's experiments and his interpretation of them were shaped at least in part by Darwin's writings on evolution, although it is also clear that

---

*An excellent discussion of the influence of Mendel's education and cultural background on his work can be found at R. Blumberg's web site http://www.netspace.org/MendelWeb. The hypertext associations are especially useful.

Mendel began his analysis of heredity in plant hybrids well before Darwin's *Origin of Species* was published in 1859. An understanding of the inheritance of biological characteristics was crucial to Darwin's evolutionary theory, which was ultimately based on the production, transmission, and environmental selection of new and different biological traits. Darwin in fact generated his own theory of heredity, which was received very seriously by the scientific community (given its source) and extensively debated, but which turned out in the fullness of time simply to be wrong.

In an appendix to Volume two of his classic work, *The Variation of Animals and Plants Under Domestication*, which appeared just two years after Mendel's paper was published, Darwin proposed that each and every part of the body produces minute copies of itself, which he called *gemmules*. The gemmules, he postulated, would migrate to the reproductive organs of a plant or animal, where they would be pooled and transmitted to the next generation, becoming mixed in the process with the gemmules contributed by the other parent involved in the reproductive event. Like most other biologists of his day, Darwin viewed offspring as essentially a blend of the two parental gene pools. He failed to see, as Mendel did, that heredity is unitary and atomistic, and that individual genetic traits do not blend; they simply cohabit. As Darwin himself admitted, his proposal was just an advanced formulation of the theory of *pangenesis*, first proposed by Greek thinkers such as Hippocrates and Aristotle. Like Mendel's genes, Darwin's gemmules were of course also abstract entities without a chemical or biological basis.

Although incorrect, Darwin's ideas on heredity did succeed in one important way: they stimulated other scientists to think very intensely about the biological basis of inheritance. In the course of developing his neo-pangenetic theory, Darwin had done his usual thorough job of pulling together an enormous range of available information and organizing it in a systematic and logical fashion. His evolutionary principles had taken the scientific community by storm, and a true understanding of those principles ultimately required a much more precise and detailed understanding of heredity. As biologists all over the world began pursuing that understanding, Darwin's own ideas on heredity fell by the wayside. And then suddenly, just at the turn of the century, Mendel's ideas were rediscovered.

In reality Mendel's ideas had never been completely lost. Although published in the proceedings of a relatively obscure natural history society (*Abhandlungen des naturforschenden Vereines in Brünn*), over one hundred copies of these proceedings were distributed to university libraries in the United States and in Europe. From time to time in the closing decades of the nineteenth century references to Mendel's paper would appear, both in scientific journals and in letters exchanged among other biologists, although it is clear from what they had to say that these biologists did not really understand the importance of what Mendel had uncovered. Part of the problem was that Mendel's approach was more mathematical and physical than many biologists were used to; part was that he carried out his work in a monastery, far from the emerging intellectual centers of his day. He seems not to have been swept up in the many exciting issues outside of heredity that were rapidly changing not just the face but the very foundations of biology. For the most part this was happening in the great universities of Europe and America, not in monasteries. This may be why Mendel never related his findings to the larger issues in the biological sciences that were engaging his contemporaries around the world; he was probably marginally aware of them at best.

In the late 1890s two botanists, Carl Correns in Germany and Hugo deVries in Holland, had independently carried out breeding experiments in plants and come to conclusions similar to Mendel's thirty-five years earlier. Just prior to publishing their own findings, each became aware of the work of Mendel through colleagues. Both acknowledged Mendel's earlier work in their own papers, published beginning in 1900. DeVries, after summarizing his own findings in the form of two "statements," said "These two statements, in their most essential points, were drawn up long ago by Mendel for a special case (peas). These formulations have been forgotten and their significance misunderstood." In a footnote, he went on to say that "[Mendel's] important treatise is so seldom cited that I first learned of its existence only after I had completed the majority of my experiments and had deduced from them the statements in the text." Correns went so far as to title his own paper "G. Mendel's Law Concerning the Behavior of Progeny of Varietal Hybrids" and declared that "Mendel's paper . . . is among the best that has ever been written about hybrids. . . . " (Mendel's work was also discovered in 1900 by a third botanist, Erich Tschermak, but it is not obvious from what he wrote that Tschermak actually understood Mendel's analysis.)

Within a very short time Mendel, who died in 1884, went from obscurity to renown; his ideas were discussed extensively in the most progressive research centers of the day, capturing the imagination in particular of the younger generation of scientists eager to upset the staid and generally unproductive approaches of their mentors. In pursuing the molecular basis of Mendel's observations, science and medicine would arrive together at the gates of molecular medicine and gene therapy. Mendel's contributions to biology are now recognized as being every bit as important as those of Darwin, in whose great shadow Mendel labored and where he was, for a time, lost.

Germ Cells and Chromosomes

The great seventeenth-century English physician-scientist William Harvey is best known for his 1628 publication of a paper showing that the heart functions as a pump to drive the blood throughout the body by way of arteries. But, in his 1651 publication, "The Generation of Animals," Harvey proposed an equally radical and profound, if initially less noticed, idea: that *all* animals — not just the chickens that were his primary object of study — originate from an egg or *ovum* produced by the female of the species. The origin of embryos had long been a matter of wild speculation: ideas had ranged from spontaneous generation in the womb to condensation from unsloughed menstrual blood. Harvey did not believe that embryos could arise from unaltered ova alone. He was of course aware of the obligatory role of the male in reproduction, but was unsure of exactly what males contributed. The early microscopist Anton van Leeuwenhoek was the first to describe, in 1677, *spermatozoa* in the semen of male animals and humans. He even postulated (albeit with no evidence) that these tiny "sperm animals" might play a role in impregnation of the female. Over the next two hundred years the concept gradually developed, largely under the influence of these two highly influential thinkers and their followers, that the reproduction of a human being involves an initial activation of an ovum by a male sperm. Sperm and ova quickly came to be regarded as the most likely vehicles for transmission of inherited traits from one generation to the next.

The exact nature of sperm and ova did not become clear until the middle of the nineteenth century, with the advent of the *cell theory*. In the 1840s two German biologists, Matthias Schleiden and Theodor

Schwann, proposed that all plants and animals are composed of large numbers of microscopic, autonomous units of life, called cells. (Cells were so-called because to early microscopists these structural units of tissue, particularly in plants, looked like rows of monk's cells in a monastery dormitory.) Cells had first been described by van Leeuwenhoek, among others, but their functional significance was not clear until Schleiden and Schwann proposed the cell theory. Over the next twenty years it was established that every tissue in the body, including the gonads, is indeed composed of living cells. The cellular nature of ova was immediately obvious, but it took somewhat longer to establish that the strangely shaped sperm were also cells. The physical union of sperm and ova during *fertilization* was first observed in 1854 by George Newport in his studies of frog reproduction.

Thus by the time genes were identified conceptually in the closing decades of the nineteenth century, it was assumed that sperm and ova (*germ cells*) would be the most likely repository for them. But where inside the germ cells would genes be stored? What would they be made of, and how would they work? The first discrete substructure, or *organelle*, to be identified inside of cells was the nucleus. Because nuclei are quite large, they can often be seen in cells using even relatively crude microscopes. In fact the nucleus was soon taken to be the one unambiguous structure defining a cell in both animals and plants. (Obviously this definition would not work in bacterial cells, which have no nucleus. But the tiny bacteria were not identified in the microscope for many years after plant and animal cells were first discovered.)

Indirect evidence had already suggested the nucleus as the portion of the cell most likely to control reproduction and heredity. For example, experiments had shown that certain very large single-cell organisms can be cut in half without killing them. The nucleus itself was not divided, so only one of the two halves of the cell ended up with a nucleus. It was observed that only the portion of the cell retaining an intact nucleus was able to reproduce itself.

During the 1880s, a remarkable series of experiments carried out by biologists in Germany provided strong evidence that the nuclear components controlling heredity are the highly specialized structures called *chromosomes*. Chromosomes had first been described in 1873 by Friedrich Schneider simply as a mass of fibers associated with the nucleus during cell division. As the cell prepared to divide, the nucleus itself seemed to disappear, and the fibers seemed to emerge out of nowhere. The fibers then lined up parallel to one another and partitioned themselves into the two newly forming daughter cells. The daughter cells would soon reform a nucleus, but then the fibers could no longer be seen. This process seemed so bizarre that neither Schneider nor anyone else knew what to make of it at first. The only time the fibers could be seen was at the time of cell division. Were they special structures that formed simply to help the cell divide, and then disappeared? If not, where were they when the cell was not actively dividing?

Although difficult to observe even at the time of cell division, Schneider's fibers turned out to be very real indeed. As the quality of microscopes improved, anyone who looked carefully enough at a dividing cell could see them. A careful study of the nuclear events accompanying cell division, which came to be called *mitosis*, was published by Walther Flemming in 1882. Flemming had been among the leaders in using various chemical stains and dyes to visualize more clearly the detailed antomy of cells, particularly the nucleus. The nucleus was known to contain a mixture of two kinds of biological molecules, protein and nucleic acid called *nuclein* at the time. Because of its strong staining properties, Flemming coined the term *chromatin* for this mixture from the Greek *chroma*, meaning "color." He showed that chromatin was present in the nuclei of cells at all stages of the cell cycle, not only at cell division. Just as a cell prepares to enter mitosis, the chromatin, which had been dispersed throughout the nucleus between cell divisions (and hence difficult to see) condenses into threadlike fibers that ultimately came to be called chromosomes.

As shown in Figure 1-3, chromosomes go through a precisely regulated sequence of steps in connection with cell division. In Figure 1-3a, a parental nucleus containing two representative chromosomes is shown; one member of each pair was inherited from the mother, and one from the father. Just prior to cell division, each chromosome is reproduced exactly; the chromosome "twins" are connected at a special structure found on each chromosome called the centromere (Figure 1-3b). The nuclei at this stage are said to be *tetraploid* in terms of DNA content. In the final stages of mitosis, as the daughter cells begin to separate from one another in cell division, one member of each twinned pair goes to the nucleus of each of the new daughter cells. The result is daughter nuclei

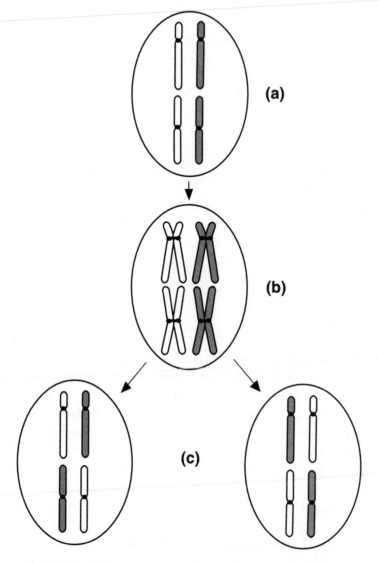

Figure 1-3. Doubling and redistribution of DNA during normal cell division (mitosis).

(Figure 1-3c) that are again diploid and genotypically identical to the parental nucleus.

Subsequent work by Flemming and his followers also showed that a normal set of chromosomes was itself double, or *diploid*; a cell normally carries (and passes on to each daughter cell at mitosis) two copies of each distinct chromosome. The fact that all living cells are diploid — ie have two copies of every gene — has important implications for genetic disease and for gene therapy. In almost all cases, a single good copy of a gene is sufficient to maintain biological function. That means that in order for an animal to suffer from a genetic deficiency, *both* copies of a given gene must be defective. That is the main reason that genetic diseases are relatively rare. But since one copy of a gene is usually sufficient for function, we do not have to repair nature's mistake fully; it is enough to replace or repair only one of the defective genes.

Flemming's observations on the replication of chromosomes and their distribution into daughter cells applied to all cells in the body, not just to germ cells. Yet at this stage in the birth of the field of genetics, genes were thought of mostly in terms of heredity and thus associated explicitly with germ cells. Could the chromosomes be the actual physical structure with which the heritable genes are associated? One peculiarity of germ cells described by Oskar Hertwig in 1876 suggested that chromosomes were indeed the vehicles of heredity and the bearer of genes. Hertwig showed that shortly after a sperm and ovum unite in fertilization to form a *zygote* (the embryo before the first embryonic cell division has taken place), the nuclei contributed by the sperm and ovum (called the *pronuclei*) fuse to form the first embryonic nucleus.

It was gradually recognized that if the chromosomes within these nuclei are indeed the bearers of heredity, then they would have to carry not a diploid set of chromosomes, but a *haploid* set, a single copy of each chromosome rather than a pair. For if both pronuclei were diploid, then after fusion the first zygotic nucleus (and all subsequent embryonic nuclei) would be tetraploid. When these tetraploid embryos reached adulthood and mated, their offspring would be octaploid, and so on. Thus August Weismann predicted in 1887 that germ cells should be haploid rather than diploid (although this prediction was clearly implicit in Mendel's model twenty years earlier). Within a short time it was established that germ cells do indeed undergo a special type of cell division (*meiosis*) in which the final number of chromosomes in their nuclei is reduced by half to make them haploid. As shown in Figure 1-4, the initial stages of meiosis, which occurs only in germ cells, are similar to mitosis, resulting in transiently connected pairs of twinned chromosomes. However, during meiosis, the newly twinned chromosomes derived from

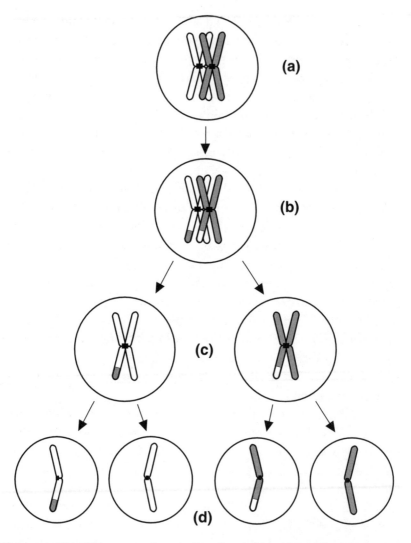

Figure 1-4. The DNA content of germ cell nuclei is halved and recombined during meiosis.

the mother physically associate with the matching pair from the father, allowing the exchange ("crossing over") of small portions of homologous chromosomes (Figure 1-4b). After this step, the germ cells divide to produce a first set of diploid daughter nuclei with newly recombined chromosome pairs (Figure 1-4c). Note that these recombined chromosomes per se did not exist in the original parental phenotype (Figure 1-4a). In the final stage of meiosis, these daughters divide again to produce germ cells that are haploid, and have a random mixture of paternal and maternal chromosomes, some of which have been recombined.

By the early 1900s, the evidence was overwhelming, albeit indirect, that the behavior of chromosomes during reproduction parallels exactly the known behavior of Mendel's genes. In a 1903 paper titled "The Chromosomes in Heredity," Walter Sutton took the leap: he proposed that Mendel's genes were a physical part of chromosomes. Each cell in a given organism has a defined set of chromosomes housing its genes. This set consists of two copies of each chromosome, one inherited from the father, and one from the mother. The germ cells, because of meiosis, contain only one copy of each chromosome. Each of the different chromosomes in a germ cell can come from either the mother or the father; the determination is random. It is during meiosis that separately inherited alleles, which Mendel had shown always remained separate and distinct, go their separate ways into different germ cells.

This physical picture of inheritance holds true today essentially as Sutton proposed it in the early years of the twentieth century. There was one immediate consequence for Mendel's views of heredity, however: the number of chromosomes observed in cells varies from a few to a few dozen. Unquestionably, if genes are to control the inheritance and expression of every single feature of a plant or animal, then the number of genes must be considerably larger than the number of chromosomes. This means that each chromosome must house many genes, necessitating the concept of *gene linkage*. Although the segregation of chromosomes into germ cells is completely random, if we follow the fate of individual genes we see that this is not always so. All of the genes of a given chromosome are said to be linked, such that where one goes, barring crossing over events, they all must go. Thus the majority of the independently segregating genes followed by Mendel in experiments of the type shown in Figure 1-2 must have resided on separate chromosomes.

Within a few years of the "rediscovery" of Mendel and the establishment of chromosomes as the physical locus of genes, it was realized that the genes Mendel had defined in terms of inheritance in plants were also responsible for inheritance in animals, including humans. The set of chromosomes containing the human *genome* is shown in Figure 1-5. This apparent unity and universality of the principles of heredity opened up

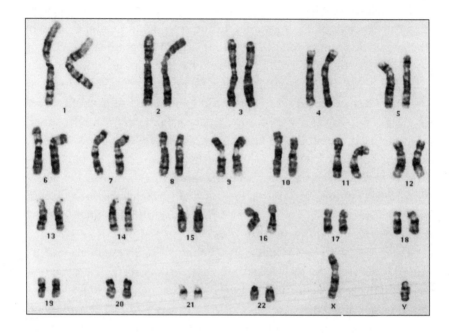

Figure 1-5. The complete set of human chromosomes. Humans have 46 chromosomes, comprising twenty-two pairs of matched *autosomes* (numbered arbitrarily 1–22), and two *sex chromosomes*, called X and Y. Males have an X and a Y chromosome in addition to the twenty-two pairs of autosomes; females have two X chromosomes. Each chromosome is composed of a thread of DNA, which contains all the genes. (The complete collection of genes and associated DNA, described in more detail in Chapters 3 and 5, is referred to as the human *genome*.) Each chromosome also has associated with it numerous proteins, which provide most of the bulk, and take up various chemical stains to produce distinct chromosomal *bands*. These bands are always the same from individual to individual, and thus provide useful landmarks for identifying specific regions associated with each chromosome. (Courtesy Dr. Robert Sparkes, Department of Medicine, UCLA.)

one of the most fruitful and dynamic lines of inquiry in the history of biology. Thus was founded the field of *genetics*, which took its name formally in 1906.

The Chemical Basis of Heredity

One of the major milestones in the evolution of scientific thought was surely the realization, which emerged gradually throughout the nineteenth century, that biological organisms—including human beings—are governed by the same laws that apply to the rest of the physical universe. The idea that humans are somehow special and apart from the rest of creation would probably have seemed strange to many earlier peoples—the ancient Greeks, for example—but came to permeate Western thinking in most of the past two millennia. Attempts to promote a humbler view of human beings were strongly resisted; nowhere was this more true than in the field of chemistry. The notion that life has a chemical basis, and that the chemical reactions taking place in a plant or animal obey the same rules as chemical reactions in the laboratory, was a revolution in human thought that can scarcely be underestimated. But by the beginning of the twentieth century, this point of view was firmly in place within the general scientific community. An attempt to understand biology within the context of chemistry led naturally to the formation of an entirely new discipline that came to be known as *biochemistry*.

Although our physical world is composed of a hundred or so naturally occurring chemical atoms, it turns out that the molecules used to generate and sustain life are made almost entirely from only six of these atoms: carbon, hydrogen, oxygen, nitrogen, sulfur and phosphorus (in chemical shorthand: C, H, O, N, S, and P, respectively). Early biochemists realized that many of the atoms of living organisms are organized into very large and complex structures found only in plants and animals; they called these structures *biological macromolecules*. By the mid-1860s, three major groups of macromolecules had been identified: *proteins*, which would turn out to be polymers of the smaller *amino acids*; *carbohydrates*, which include the simple sugars and the more complex starches; and *lipids*, which include the water-insoluble fats.

The fourth and final major group of biological macromolecules, the *nucleic acids*, was first described at the very end of the 1860s by Johann Friedrich Miescher, a young Swiss scientist studying with the great German chemist Ernst Hoppe-Seyler in Tübingen. At Hoppe-Seyler's urging, Miescher began trying to work out the biochemistry of the cell nucleus, working with white blood cells isolated from pus adhering to surgical bandages. The nuclei in these cells proved relatively easy to isolate, enabling him to study their contents more or less uncontaminated by other cellular components. The material inside the nuclei appeared to be macromolecular in nature, but the phosphorus content was considerably higher—two to three percent overall—than any of the three known biochemical groups. Convinced that he had discovered a new category of biological macromolecules, Miescher called the new substance *nuclein*, in recognition of its origin.

Upon returning to Switzerland in 1874, Miescher turned to a more practical source of nuclein. His institute in Basel was near the headwaters of the Rhine, which at that time was well stocked with salmon. Salmon sperm turned out to be an excellent source of nuclei (in fact a sperm is mostly a nucleus, surrounded by very little other cellular material), and the supply was almost endless, at least in summer. (Thanks largely to Miescher's work, salmon sperm remains to this day one of the most common sources of DNA for general experimental purposes.) Miescher soon realized that nuclein was not a pure substance, but rather a complex of protein, which had no detectable phosphorus, with an acidic molecule of even higher phosphorus content, which he estimated to be around five percent. This new substance (which in its purest form turns out to have a phosphorus content closer to ten percent) came to be known as *nucleic acid*. Eventually, it was realized that nucleic acid from the nucleus is one of two major classes of nucleic acid. Nuclear nucleic acid is called *deoxyribonucleic acid* or DNA. A second class of nucleic acid, called *ribonucleic acid* (RNA) has a slightly different chemical composition. It is found both in the nucleus and in the *cytoplasm* (the viscous sap constituting the non-nuclear portions of the cell), and serves a variety of functions in the cell distinct from DNA. We will examine some of the functions of RNA in a subsequent chapter.

Neither Miescher nor anyone else at the time had the slightest idea of the function of nucleic acids. The mystery only deepened when DNA proved to be a polymer formed from basic building blocks called *nucleotides* (Figure 1-6). Each nucleotide consists of a central base, and a five-carbon sugar molecule with a highly oxygenated phosphorous atom (a *phosphate group*) attached. There are only four different bases used

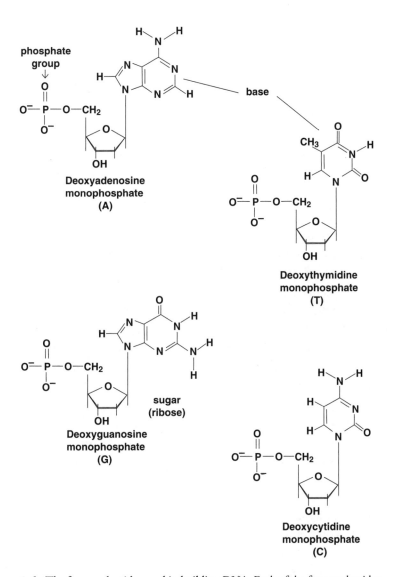

Figure 1-6. The four nucleotides used in building DNA. Each of the four nucleotides shown are usually referred to by their abbreviations: A, T, G, and C. All four nucleotides have in common a phosphate group, and a 5-membered sugar (ribose) ring. Each nucleotide is distinguished by a unique *base* composed of either one or two nitrogen-containing rings.

in DNA, with the same sugar phosphate attached; the four resulting nucleotides are called *adenosine*, *thymidine*, *guanosine*, and *cytidine* (referred to by biochemists simply as A, T, G, and C; see Figure 1-6.) DNA is nothing more than an enormous linear polymer of what appeared for many years to be random groupings of these four nucleotides.

By the early 1900s it was clear that chromosomes and chromatin were identical, and that chromatin was in turn simply Miescher's nuclein, a mixture of protein and nucleic acid (DNA). The evidence that chromosomes were also the carriers of Mendel's genes was by then indisputable. The profound implication of this was apparent early on to American biologist E. B. Wilson, who stated in an 1895 paper: "And thus we reach the remarkable conclusion that inheritance may, perhaps, be effected by the physical transmission of a particular chemical compound from parent to offspring." This hypothesis turned out to be absolutely true. Acceptance of this idea did not come easily; for those who found the concept that life itself had a chemical basis disturbing, the notion that something as mysterious and elusive as heredity could also be purely chemical in nature would prove extremely difficult to embrace. Could genes really be just another kind of chemistry?

Two key questions would occupy geneticists for the next half century: "What exactly are genes?" and "How do genes work?" More than one Nobel Prize would be earned on the way to answering these questions. We will continue to trace the thread of basic research accompanying this quest, because a true understanding of molecular medicine — both its promises and its pitfalls — depends on a solid grasp of molecular genetics.

But first, let us begin to explore some of the diseases — and the genes involved — upon which molecular medicine and gene therapy are likely to have a major impact. We will look at four diseases in all. Two — cystic fibrosis and severe combined immune deficiency (SCID) — are diseases of children, and are caused by defects in single genes. Molecular medicine is being used to treat these two diseases by gene therapy — the introduction of normal copies of the affected genes into living cells within the body. Two other diseases, cancer and AIDS, affect both children and adults. Cancer usually involves multiple gene mutations in its victims. AIDS does not involve mutated genes at all; it is caused by an invading virus. Clinical trials are currently underway for these two diseases as well;

in these cases molecular medicine will be used to introduce genes that will alter or destroy the affected cells. A close look at all four diseases, and what has happened so far in applying the techniques of molecular medicine to their treatment, will provide us with a window to the future of medicine in the twenty-first century.

2

Cystic Fibrosis

Cystic fibrosis (CF) is a terrible disease because it strikes children and because there is no cure. It is caused by a defect in one of Mendel's "atoms of heredity," a tiny mistake in a single gene. CF has obviously been a disease in the human population for a very long time; people suffering from symptoms associated with CF (such as excessively salty sweat preceding or accompanying a serious illness) have been described in the medical literature for at least several hundred years. But a precise clinical definition of CF did not emerge until the late 1930s. Dr. Dorothy Andersen, a pathologist at Columbia University, had become intrigued by several cases of newborns, infants, and children she had seen at autopsy that seemed to share certain symptoms. Comparing these with other cases gleaned from the medical literature, she felt she could fit them together into a common syndrome, implying the possibility of a single underlying cause.

In 1938 Andersen published a landmark paper in which she described in detail the cases of forty-nine such children, aged three days to fourteen years. Five of these young patients had died within the first week of life from intestinal obstruction. Nineteen died within the first six months of life, with the remainder dying between six months and fourteen years. All had one thing in common: when examined under the microscope, their pancreases were full of dense, functionless clots of scarlike tissue. She thus termed the condition "cystic fibrosis of the pancreas." However, all of the patients succumbing after the first few weeks of life actually died of degenerative lung disease characterized by extensive bacterial infection, and not of pancreatic complications. In her initial paper, Andersen did not speculate about how a problem in the pancreas could result in lung disease. This far-ranging nature of the CF defect creates difficulties both for diagnosis (it is often confused initially with pneumonia or asthma) and for treatment.

As often happens when a new disease is first described, based on a thoughtful analysis of scientific and clinical data, Andersen's report triggered an avalanche in the medical journals of previously unreported cases that clearly fit the syndrome. Recognition that these superficially unrelated symptoms could have a common origin, that they could be caused by a single physiological defect, was an important first step. For several years, most research into CF was directed toward developing a more complete picture of this disease both clinically and pathologically. Then came the question of treatment. From the very beginning, each of the problems associated with CF—respiratory distress, pancreatic insufficiency, intestinal problems—has had to be treated as if it were a separate disease. No one knew what tied them together. With time, and a great deal of clinical experimentation, the outlook for children with CF gradually improved, but it remains to this day one of the most intractable of childhood illnesses.

A few decades ago, children with the more severe forms of CF rarely lived to school age. Although many now survive well into the third decade of life, the quality of these added years is not always good. The normal pressures of adolescence for the child with CF are magnified many times over by the stigma of being burdened with "a disease", and the sense of being unattractive or undesirable to the opposite sex. As they become young adults, the knowledge that they are unable to have children of their own compounds their sense of inadequacy, but worst of all is the gradual understanding that their lives will be drastically foreshortened. By the third decade of life, increasingly frequent hospitalizations put tremendous emotional pressure on both the patient and the family. Both know that one day, one of these visits will be the last.

To truly understand what is wrong in CF, we must first understand a little about *epithelial ducts* and the cells that line them. Epithelial ducts are like tunnels. Imagine driving through a tunnel passing beneath a river. The purpose of the tunnel is to get us from one side of the river to the other without contaminating us with the surrounding mud and water, and to deliver us to a precise point on the other side of the river without floating off to unintended places downstream. Ducts do the same thing inside the body; they allow rapid and precise delivery of substances from one place to another without contamination by surrounding material, and without spilling these substances out into the general circulation.

The human body is full of such ducts. The pancreas and the liver have ducts into which they pour enzymes and other substances that travel to the intestines to help digest food. The lungs are full of epithelium-lined passages (the *bronchi* and *bronchioles*) for taking in and expelling air. The female breast has special ducts to gather milk and deliver it to the nipple during nursing. Like tunnels, which are often lined with geometric tiles to provide a smooth inner surface, the inner surface of ducts are lined with tilelike *epithelial cells*. But ducts have an additional lining, a coating of slimy, jellylike material called *mucus* overlaying the epithelial cells. Imagine that the tunnel we are driving through has a coating of thickish, transparent Jell-o smeared over all the tiles. Like Jell-o, mucus is made of protein and sugar dissolved or suspended in water. The protein and sugar portions of mucus are made by special cells scattered throughout the epithelial lining called *goblet cells*, and by special mucus-secreting glands located just below the epithelial layer.

Mucus plays a variety of different roles, depending on the epithelial surface with which it is associated. In the gut, it acts as a lubricant to smooth the passage of food, and to protect the intestinal epithelial cells from damage caused by bone fragments, sharp seeds, or other indigestible material. Mucus can also make it difficult for bacteria or other microbes to penetrate into the body across epithelial surfaces. This is particularly important in the nose, throat, and lungs, where airborne microbes are taken in with virtually every breath. Mucus is a naturally sticky substance that readily traps anything coming into the airway. Microscopic hairlike structures called *cilia* line many epithelial surfaces. These cilia beat in synchrony—much like a "wave" passing around a sports stadium—just below the mucus layer, pushing along the mucus and any material trapped in it in a slowly moving stream. Most particulate matter coming in through the nose, for example, is trapped by nasal hairs and rides on a wave of cilia-driven mucus into the throat and then the stomach, where it is destroyed.

Mucus is at the heart of the defect in CF. In order for it to function properly, mucus must be of a certain thickness, or *viscosity*. Viscosity is critical both in lubrication and in entrapment of particulate matter. The viscosity of mucus is controlled largely by its water content, and this is the source of the problem in CF patients. Production of the protein and sugar portions of mucus appears to be perfectly normal, but not enough water gets mixed into it. As a result, the mucus lining all of the epithelial ducts throughout the body is simply too thick. It does not move along on the underlying cilia; it accumulates and may eventually completely block the duct. As we shall see, correcting this inability to properly *hydrate* (secrete water into) mucus is the target of CF gene therapy.

In the lungs, the accumulation of thick mucus in airways causes two problems. First, clots of mucus can impede the passage of air, particularly expelled air. When we breathe in, muscles in the chest pull the air in; the more we contract these muscles, the more air we take in. CF patients can compensate for partially blocked airways simply by breathing in harder. Breathing out, on the other hand, is different; there are no muscles we can use to force the air out. Exhaling involves simply a relaxation of the muscles used to bring air in. Thus CF patients, like asthmatics, often have lungs hyperinflated with stale, oxygen-poor air.

The second and more serious problem is that the thickened mucus becomes infected with bacteria and other pathogens in inhaled air. The most common infections involve *Staphylococcus aureus, Pseudomonas aeruginosa,* and *Hemophilus influenza. Pseudomonas* is what gives CF mucus its characteristic green color. Mucus is a normal part of the defense against such pathogens, and their presence triggers the production of even more mucus, compounding the problem. The lungs are equipped with powerful immune defenses that ordinarily clear away these and other pathogens quickly as they try to penetrate through the mucus into the underlying epithelium. But the immobilized clots of stagnant mucus provide a breeding ground for pathogens that is difficult for the immune system to deal with. It is very difficult for the cells and molecules of the immune system to penetrate the thickened mucus to get at the pathogens.

Nevertheless, they keep trying and, in attempting to clear the infected mucus away, a process called *inflammation* is set in motion.

Inflammation is a violent, all-out attack on foreign invaders that can cause serious damage to nearby healthy cells and tissues. Most inflammatory reactions are shortlived; the infection is cleared away and the immune cells leave the area after producing chemicals that initiate a healing process. But in chronic inflammation the destruction continues unabated, as does the toll on the surrounding healthy tissue. In the airways and lungs of CF patients, the loss of tissue greatly compounds the loss of function caused by clogging with overly thick mucus. A combination of these two defects leads to one of the earliest diagnostic features in young CF patients: a persistent, increasingly harsh cough accompanied by expectoration of thick, greenish phlegm. The cycles of infection, tissue destruction, and ductal obstruction continue until the lungs can no longer take in enough oxygen to support the needs of the rest of the body. Activity is slowed, and appetite decreases. Eventually the patient dies of *anoxia* (lack of oxygen). Current treatments, centered on the use of antibiotics and teaching the patient and family members how to dislodge clogged mucus, have definitely contributed to prolonging the life of CF patients.

A similar problem also occurs in the pancreas. The pancreas has two quite distinct functions. One subset of cells (comprising the *endocrine* portion of the pancreas) produces the hormones insulin and glucagon for general release into the bloodstream. These cells are largely unaffected in CF, at least in the early stages of the disease. The majority of the pancreatic cells, however, make enzymes used to digest food and comprise the *exocrine* pancreas. These digestive enzymes are released into epithelial ducts for transport to the small intestine just at the point where it leaves the stomach. The thickened mucus present in all epithelial ducts in CF patients eventually blocks these exocrine ducts, and the digestive enzymes cannot reach the intestines. This is the aspect of CF first noted by Dorothy Andersen in 1938. As a result of the blockage, the ability to digest food is greatly impaired; CF patients are constantly hungry and eat large quantities of food, yet they remain undernourished and fail to grow normally. Vitamins that are dissolved in the fatty portions of food are not released properly for absorption through the intestine because fats are not properly digested. Youngsters often experience chronic diarrhea. Because of the poor digestion, the stools are fatty and foul smelling, and malodorous flatulence is a distressing social problem for many CF patients throughout life. By the time CF patients succumb to lung disease, they have lost nearly all of the enzyme function of their pancreas. In advanced stages of the disease, the fibrotic exocrine tissue may even begin to press in on the endocrine portion of the pancreas and interfere with insulin production, leading to a form of diabetes.

In about ten percent of CF patients, an intestinal blockage by mucus at the time of birth can be fatal if not treated immediately. As food comes into the newborn's system for the first time, it pushes the dark green, mucus-containing contents of the fetal intestines (called *meconium*) ahead for elimination by normal defecation. In affected CF infants, the meconium is too thick for normal passage through the intestinal tract. Digestive enzymes from the pancreas normally help clear meconium from the system, but in these infants the pancreas may already be fibrotic, and not enough enzymes reach the intestine. At some point the meconium stops moving, and that region of the intestine (usually the ileum) begins to swell. As oncoming meconium and food wastes pile up behind the initial meconium block, distention continues. The infant often vomits repeatedly. The inflated intestine may begin to wrap around itself, crimping the blood supply and causing gangrene. If this condition is not corrected by surgery or other means within a day or two, the intestines may burst, which can be fatal. Problems related to bowel function are also not uncommon in older CF patients, but the consequences are not usually so deadly.

Over the years, improvements in the treatment of the various manifestations of CF have greatly extended survival for affected children, but in the past decade additional gains have been minimal. This may indicate that current approaches to managing CF are close to optimal based on the available technology. Problems with digestion can be managed reasonably well by giving the enzymes lost from the pancreas in tablet form, with a special coating that allows the enzymes to pass unharmed through the strong acid of the stomach and into the intestine where they are needed. Even with this added help, however, digestion and utilization of food is less than optimal, so patients are kept on a high-calorie diet with extra doses of most vitamins. Fat-soluble vitamins are given in particular excess to compensate for their poor absorption rate.

Congested airways can be cleared to some extent by physical means such as vigorous clapping on the back and chest while coughing and expectorating. This may need to be done several times as day, and can obviously be uncomfortable for the patient. Vigorous exercise can also be of some help in bringing up excess mucus. Bronchodilators such as those used for asthma are occasionally useful in keeping airways open. Very recently drugs have become available that appear to help thin out the mucus. One, interestingly, works on DNA. As part of the inflammatory process, various white blood cells are attracted to the pathogen-loaded mucus, where they attempt to clear the infection. In the process, many of the white cells die, spilling their DNA into the area. DNA itself is very thick and sticky, compounding the general problem. The enzyme *DNAse*, which digests DNA, clears away the DNA and apparently reduces clogging significantly. How effective such drugs will be in the longterm remains to be seen.

Infection by bacterial pathogens remains a problem; antibiotics were important in extending lifespan when first used for treating CF patients, but unfortunately the rate of discovery of new, more effective antibiotics has slowed greatly. Moreover, some antibiotics must be given by injection or by intravenous drip at least once and often several times a day. Patient compliance is a constant problem. Lung infection and destruction is by far the most deadly aspect of CF, and repair of the CF defect in lung and airway tissue is the immediate goal of CF gene therapy.

The Cystic Fibrosis Gene

CF is one of the most common genetic diseases in the United States, accounting for more deaths each year than any other inherited disease. CF is caused by a defect in a single gene; we know this because of the strict Mendelian pattern of inheritance. The underlying defect, like the "wrinkled" trait in peas, is recessive — that is, a defect must occur in *both* inherited copies of the affected gene. Both parents of a CF child must therefore be heterozygotes or *carriers*, each parent "carrying" one good gene and one defective gene. Heterozygotes are perfectly normal in every way — apparently one good copy of the CF gene is enough to get along on. Just as predicted from Mendel's study in peas, on average one child in four of heterozygous carrier parents will be homozygous for the defective gene; he or she will have CF. One child in four will also, on average, have two good copies of the CF gene. And two children in four will be perfectly healthy heterozyous carriers like their parents. As we shall see, recent advances in the molecular biology of CF have made it possible to identify the exact genetic status of each individual in families affected by CF. This information will allow unaffected children of CF-heterozygous parents to plan their own reproductive futures in a more informed way. (CF children are almost always sterile as adults.)

CF is especially devastating in the Caucasian population: one in twenty Caucasians are estimated to be carriers of a defective CF gene, with a somewhat lower frequency among Hispanics and a negligible frequency among African Americans. As many as one in two thousand Caucasian infants are born with CF. Why the frequency for such a deadly gene should be at such a high level in the general population is something of a mystery. One might reasonably expect that a gene that, as recently as fifty years ago, killed the vast majority of its victims before reproductive age would have nearly disappeared from the species by now. Some have speculated that a defective CF gene in heterozygotes may somehow confer protection to some other deadly disease. Overall, one child with CF is born per 3,000 live births each year in the U.S., which translates into about 1,300 new cases per year. A few dozen more die in the womb. Boys and girls are affected equally. There are over 30,000 CF patients currently alive in the U.S. alone, but the average life expectancy for these people is still under thirty years.

Numerous experiments were carried out in the 1960s and 1970s to try to understand the biochemical basis of the CF defect. There are many possible explanations for the accumulation of thickened mucus in epithelial ducts; any reasonable mechanism that was put forward was thoroughly investigated, but for many years there were no definitive results. Many diseases in humans have their counterpart in a disease occuring naturally in animals, the so-called "animal models" for human disease. Often, rapid progress toward understanding the origin and basis of a given human disease can be made by studying animal models, and applying the results, with suitable modifications, to humans. Unfortunately, no animal model for CF was ever uncovered. It had become clear by the 1980s that further progress in understanding and treating CF would require a definitive description of the defect involved in humans, and that the best way to get this information would be to use recently developed technology for isolating the CF gene itself and to study the gene directly. Moreover, because CF is clearly caused by a single defective gene, isolating and cloning the gene would open up the posibility of gene therapy, which, by the mid-1980s, was on the minds of everyone working on genetically based diseases.

By 1986, using techniques of both classical and molecular genetics to follow the inheritance of the CF gene in affected families, researchers had traced the location of the gene to human chromosome seven and the gene was found to map to a specific position on this chromosome. These classical genetic mapping studies were a tour de force occupying a number of laboratories for at least a decade. But each human chromosome contains a huge amount of genetic information; what may appear like a tiny point on a drawing of a chromosome may still contain an enormous number of genes. An enormous number, but not an impossible number.

The hunt for the actual CF gene began in earnest in the mid 1980s. A different set of research laboratories took over from the chromosome mappers, and began applying the latest techniques of molecular biology with massive force. There was a definite feeling that it could be done, that the gene could be found. The prize was huge; to be the first to identify the gene responsible for such a devastating disease could secure the reputations of scientists and institutions alike. Moreover, isolating the gene would be just the first step. Figuring out what the gene product was, and how mutations in it caused the disease, would become an exciting chase in itself. Already the gene doctors were beginning to plan exactly how they would use good copies of the gene to compensate for the bad, and bring this disease to its knees once and for all.

The identity of the gene was finally revealed in three papers published in the September 1989 issue of the journal *Science*. (We will see exactly how the CF gene was isolated in Chapter 7.) Isolating the gene was an enormous task. The *Science* papers involved twenty-four different scientists, based mostly at the Hospital for Sick Children in Toronto, but with collaborators at the University of Michigan and the University of Pennsylvania. Isolation of the CF gene was a watershed event in the history of this disease. Both patients and researchers to this day speak in terms of "before" and "after" finding the gene. The actual identity of the gene was a surprise, although once everyone knew what it encoded it seemed, in hindsight, perfectly logical.

As we have learned, the major problem in CF is excessively thick mucus in the epithelial ducts. Therefore, a candidate gene for CF must be tied in some way to mucus production. One possibility might be a gene that controls the water content, and hence the viscosity, of mucus. Water secretion from epithelial cells, which would be required to properly hydrate the mucus, has been known for many years to be largely controlled by the uptake and secretion of salt. This is an ongoing and very active process; several liters of fluids per day are secreted across the body's various epithelial surfaces. Salts—mostly sodium chloride and potassium chloride—are actively pumped back and forth across cell membranes as a part of normal cellular functions. The overall salt concentration inside a cell, however, must be kept within very strict limits, so the amount of water in the cell must always be regulated in synchrony with salt transport. For example, if salt is pumped into a cell, water must also be brought in so that the cell's overall concentration of salt does not rise too high. Accordingly, if salt is pumped out of a cell, water must accompany it so that the cell's salt concentration does not become too low (Figure 2-1).

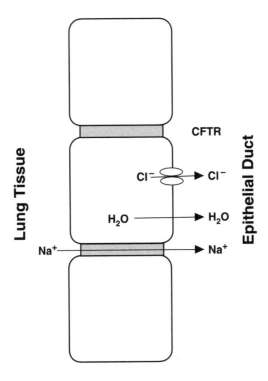

Figure 2-1. Exchange of water and salt ions across epithelial cells. Shown here schematically is a cross-section through epithelial cells such as those lining a typical epithelial duct in the lung. The opening or "lumen" of the duct is on the right hand side of the drawing, and the lung tissue through which the duct is passing is to the left. (In this cross-section only one wall of the duct is shown.)

This knowledge of how water secretion is regulated in cells focused increasing attention on defective salt pumps (or "channels," as they are called by cell biologists) as a possible source of the problem. As shown in the accompanying Figure, water is secreted by cells when chloride ions (usually accompanied by sodium ions) are pumped from epithelial cell layers into the lumen of the ducts. And that is precisely where the defect lies in CF. The gene that, when defective, causes labored breathing, blocked pancreatic ducts, defective sweat glands, impeded intestinal flow, and sterility encodes a single, membrane-associated protein called CFTR (cystic fibrosis transport regulator). Although its exact function was unclear at first, CFTR turned out to be in fact a protein that forms a chloride ion channel.

Exactly how a defective ion channel would cause the defects seen in CF is unclear, but there are several very good guesses. If the chloride channels were defective, patients would be unable to secrete water into epithelial ducts, and thickened mucus would be one result. Thickened mucus, and the entrapped bacteria, would be very difficult for the cilia to sweep into the lungs for disposal by resident scavenger cells, called *macrophages*. It is also possible that altered ionic concentrations in the epithelial lining could lead to an overproduction of mucus. Very recent laboratory results suggest that certain bactericidal (bacteria-destroying) molecules produced by normal epithelial cells are secreted in CF, but cannot function to kill bacteria in the excessively salty mucus found in CF airways. Any or all of these potential defects may be operating and could easily account for the pathology seen in the lungs of CF patients.

Once the CFTR gene was isolated and identified, physicians and scientists began comparing it among different patients. To date they have found nearly two hundred mutant forms of this gene in the CF population. This helps account for one of the disease's long-standing puzzles: although the various symptoms are almost always seen together, the relative severity of each can vary from patient to patient. Some patients barely have symptoms of the disease; others are in mortal danger from the day they are born. It is now clear that some of the observed mutations cripple the transport regulator much more seriously than do others. Working together, physicians and scientists have also found the CFTR gene to be involved in several diseases not previously connected to the CF family of disorders. For example, a sperm duct had been thought in some sterile males to be absent because of the duct's failure to develop properly in utero. This failure has now been found to be a result of a defective CFTR gene, with the same clogging, inflammation, and degeneration seen in CF patients. (Why this particular CFTR mutation affects only the sperm duct and not other tissues is unclear at present.)

What *is* the gene for CF? What does it look like? How did scientists finally find it? What is wrong with defective alleles of this gene? Most importantly, can we repair or somehow compensate for this genetic defect, and if so will this really help people with CF? To help answer these and other questions, which are at the heart of molecular medicine, let us return once more to the basic research underlying this exciting new field. If we are to understand molecular medicine, we must first understand molecular biology.

3

DNA and the Language of Genes

When E. B. Wilson suggested in 1895 that heredity might have a chemical basis, he was thinking specifically of the nucleic acid component. But this was no more than an inspired guess on his part and, indeed, of the two major components of chromatin, nucleic acid seemed to many the less likely candidate. The problem was in the perceived possibilities for information content: DNA is composed of only four basic nucleotides. The hereditary material — genes — must contain the blueprint for the construction of an entire organism. How can only four nucleotides be used to spell out the enormous complexity of a complete animal or plant? Proteins, on the other hand, are polymers of amino acids, of which there are twenty different kinds. This is close to the number of letters in most alphabets. Thus, even for scientists convinced of the chemical basis of heredity, proteins seemed intuitively to be a more likely candidate for the transmission of information from one generation to the next.

The Chemical Nature of Genes

The debate over the likely chemical nature of genes continued unresolved until the 1940s, when it was gradually put to rest through a series of elegant experiments carried out entirely in microbes. The choice of microbes for these studies was in itself revolutionary. A major realization that had made its way into scientific thinking in the early twentieth century was that not only are human beings subject to the same laws of chemistry and physics that govern the inanimate world, but that they are also constructed on a biochemical plan shared in remarkable detail with even the simplest life forms, including bacteria and funguses. Although a humbling realization, this fact, once fully understood and accepted, made it possible to carry out basic biological research highly relevant to human physiology using a wide range of inexpensive, readily obtainable microorganisms. Time and again, to the amazement of early biochemists, chemical reactions and pathways worked out in microbes (the existence of which was not even suspected just decades before) proved barely distinguishable from those defined, with considerably more difficulty, in human beings.

The first set of experiments to suggest that DNA might be the component of chromatin responsible for inheritance in living organisms involved a bacterium known as *Diplococcus pneumoniae*, which causes pneumonia in humans and mice. Different strains of this bacterium produce colonies that, under the microscope, look markedly different. Two strains in particular had attracted attention; one that made smooth colonies, and one that made rough-looking colonies. This property "bred true" from generation to generation; smooth bacteria always gave rise to smooth colonies, and rough always gave rise to rough. It was thus presumed to have a genetic basis.

When bacterial cells from smooth colonies were injected into mice at a certain dose, the mice would die of pneumonia. The same dose of cells from rough colonies had no effect on the mice. This was of great interest for obvious health reasons but, in pursuing it further, scientists made a startling and inexplicable observation. If live "rough" cells were mixed together with dead "smooth" cells, some of the rough cells began to form smooth colonies characteristic of the dead cells in the mixture. Moreover, if they were injected into mice, the previously benign rough cells would induce pneumonia in the mice and kill them.

The most likely explanation seemed that the smooth cells simply had not all been killed; no reasonable alternative interpretation could be imagined at first. So the experiment was repeated many times, with great care taken to be certain that all the smooth cells were truly dead. The results did not change. It was finally concluded that some of the rough cells had absorbed and been *transformed* by something released by the smooth-colony bacteria. Importantly, the acquisition of smoothness and the ability to cause lethal pneumonia in mice was genetically stable; once acquired, it was passed from generation to generation when the transformed bacteria divided to form new progeny.

In order to identify the transforming substance from the smooth bacteria, Oswald Avery at the Rockefeller Institute (now Rockefeller University) in New York broke open cultures of smooth bacteria, separated the cell contents into the major component biochemical groups (proteins, lipids, carbohydrates, and nucleic acids) and tested each group separately for its ability to transform rough bacteria into smooth. Only the nucleic acids had transforming power. A simple test showed that DNA, and not RNA, was the active factor.

In their landmark 1944 paper, Avery and his colleagues, echoing E. B. Wilson nearly half a century earlier, declared that the profound biological differences observed as a result of transformation represented "a change that is chemically induced and specifically directed by a chemical compound." They further speculated that "nucleic acids must be regarded as possessing biological specificity the chemical basis of which is as yet undetermined." Avery was a very careful, highly respected scientist, and not at all given to overinterpretation of his data. Nevertheless, other scientists of the time, especially those who doubted heredity could ever be chemical in the first place, argued that the establishment of DNA as the transforming factor was consistent with but did not demand that genes are themselves composed of DNA. They argued that it was theoretically possible that DNA simply caused a stable, heritable change in the genes of the transformed cells. Nevertheless, Avery's experiment caused scientists everywhere to begin an intense and critical examination of DNA as the possible substance of heredity. Prior to this experiment, no biological function had ever been ascribed to DNA. Many thought it might simply play a structural role in the chromosomes, helping them keep their characteristic rodlike shapes.

Eight years later, convincing evidence that DNA is indeed the substance of genes would be in hand and, once again, the data would come from experiments in microbes. Bacteria, like humans, are plagued by viruses. Viruses are nothing more than a piece of nucleic acid (DNA or RNA) wrapped in a thin coat of protein. They are not cells—they are not really even alive. In order to reproduce, they must make their way into a living cell and take over the cell's machinery to copy themselves. Certain particularly deadly bacterial viruses, called *bacteriophage* (literally, "bacteria eater"), or simply *phage*, infect a bacterium, shut down its activity, and use its equipment and energy stores to produce more phage. Once a hundred or so new phage have been made, they burst out through the walls of the cell like some sort of Hollywood alien, completely destroying the bacterium in the process. The new phage then invade surrounding bacteria, setting up continuing cycles of infection and destruction.

It is quite clear that the invading phage bring with them all the genetic information necessary to generate more of their own kind; this information does not reside in the bacterium. Each of these invaders will always breed true (reproduce only itself) regardless of the bacterial strain in which it reproduces. Each phage, like each living cell, contains its own built-in "substance of heredity." Since phage consist only of nucleic acid and protein, the hereditary substance must be one or the other. In a 1952 paper by Alfred Hershey and Martha Chase, it was shown that only the nucleic acid component of the phage ever enters the bacterial cell; the protein coat is left on the outside. (We now know this to be true of virtually all viruses.) It would be very difficult indeed to imagine that the protein coat of a phage, sticking to the outer surface of a bacterial cell, could orchestrate the assembly within the cell of hundreds of new phage. Having been "softened up" by Avery's experiments eight years earlier, the scientific world in the early 1950s was much more ready to be convinced that DNA was the hereditary principle. The Hershey-Chase experiment is often thought of as the turning point in the ongoing battle between those championing protein as the hereditary component of chromatin, and those believing that genes were written in the language of DNA.

At about the same time that Avery and others were coming to the conclusion that DNA is the chemical basis for genes, experiments were proceeding in other laboratories to determine exactly what it is that genes do. These experiments were carried out in yet another microorganism, this time a common mold found on stale bread, called *Neurospora crassa*. By studying carefully the consequences of genetic mutations induced in these organisms by radiation, George Beadle and Edward Tatum presented convincing evidence in 1940 that genes must encode proteins. This would turn out to be absolutely true, and was the beginning of the important genetic notion of "one gene = one protein." Proteins carry out the workaday functions of cells. Almost all of the other materials needed by the body can be made by proteins, which, in the form of enzymes, are able to promote the synthesis of all the other requisite biological molecules: carbohydrates, lipids, even DNA itself.

By the early 1950s, the evidence that heredity is chemical and that genes are composed solely of DNA and code for proteins was overwhelming. Yet two fundamental questions continued to confound even the most ardent believers in DNA: How would DNA go about reproducing itself at the start of each generation, and how could a molecule based on only four different subunits dictate the structure and function of an entire organism? Furthermore, what was the "as yet undetermined" chemical basis of biological specificity?

The way in which DNA is able to reproduce itself was revealed by James Watson's and Francis Crick's classic "thought experiments" published in two papers in the British journal *Nature* in 1953. This was one of the most exciting moments in the history of biology: it changed forever the way we think about every aspect of biology and medicine. This story has been recounted admirably in books such as Horace Freeland Judson's *Eighth Day of Creation*, or Watson's own *Double Helix*. It was through a detailed analysis of the physical structure of DNA as it exists in three-dimensional space that its mode of reproduction became apparent. The double-helical structure of DNA is shown in Figure 3-1a. Each strand of the helix is composed of a linear array of individual nucleotides (see Figure 1-6). These strands wind around each other in the by-now classic double-helix structure. The sugar and phosphate groups of individual nucleotides lie on the outside of the double-helical structure, with the bases facing inward (Figure 3-1b). Each strand has a particular reading direction, or "sense;" standard chemical notation designates a 5' (5-prime) and 3' end. Linear displays of a DNA sequence are always written in the 5' to 3' sense. The two strands are wound around each other in opposite directions, and are thus said to be *anti-parallel*. A and T always face each other, as do G and C; these pairs bond with each other and lend overall stability to the double helix. Because of this enforced and invariant pairing, the linear length of a native DNA molecule is marked off in

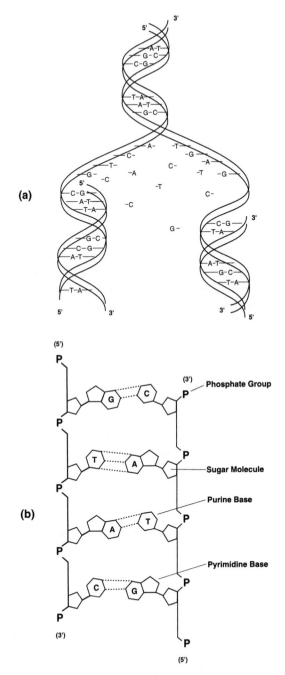

Figure 3-1. Two-dimensional representation of DNA strand interactions.

"base pairs" (bp). During mitosis or meiosis, the DNA strands in each chromosome separate, and free nucleotides present in the nucleus pair with the exposed nucleotides along each strand in accordance with the A-T, G-C rule, to form two double strands identical to the original. This process continues until the original strand is completely separated and reproduced. The new strands are incorporated into the chromosomes segregating into daughter nuclei as shown in Figures 1-3 and 1-4.

There are no chemical restrictions on the sequence of nucleotides along one DNA strand. But the sequence of nucleotides along either strand is absolutely predictable from the sequence along the opposing strand. Between any two strands of DNA, adenine (A) must always be opposite ("pair with") thymine (T); guanine (G) must always be opposite cytosine (C). It is really as simple as that. Just prior to the division of a cell, the two strands of DNA unwind from each other. Individual nucleotides assemble along each strand, obeying the A-T/G-C rule, under the influence of an enzyme called *DNA polymerase*. The nucleotides then form chemical bonds with one another to create a continuous DNA strand. At the end of this process of *DNA replication*, one DNA double helix has become two, each identical to the original. Each daughter cell thus receives a double-stranded DNA molecule identical to the one in the parental cell. This is precisely what had been predicted for the "substance of heredity" ever since the end of the nineteenth century.

This simple, elegant model — what Judson has called "a conception of astounding parsimony" — earned the Nobel Prize for its authors, and laid the groundwork for a revolution that would generate an entirely new field of scientific inquiry: molecular biology. Before that revolution could be fully realized, however, the second riddle of DNA would have to be solved: Granted that the genes written into DNA contain the instructions to make proteins, how are these instructions read? How can a cell use DNA to specify the linear amino acid sequence of a protein?

Breaking the Genetic Code

The problem of the information content of DNA was recognized as early as 1944, by the physicist Erwin Schrödinger in his highly influential book *What Is Life?*, essentially as a problem in cryptography. Schrödinger reasoned that the information contained in DNA would almost certainly be stored as a particular linear sequence of specific atomic (nucleotide) combinations. He likened this to the Morse code, where the entire English alphabet can be spelled out using only dots and dashes. By grouping the dots and dashes into clusters of three or four to represent individual letters, it is possible to spell out any message in the English (or any other alphabet-based) language. Schrödinger's speculation that nucleotide sequences in DNA could be used to direct the construction of other biological macromolecules was remarkably close to the truth. Although his book was widely read, his ideas on the problem that would become known as the *genetic code* did not seem to influence many of the people who would later work directly on the problem. Too many pieces of the puzzle were still missing to allow the leap in thinking that Schrödinger was proposing.

Ten years later, mounting indirect evidence had led almost everyone to accept that the linear sequence of nucleotides in DNA must in fact dictate the linear sequence of amino acids in protein. But this concept, logical as it might seem, still lacked any sort of direct experimental validation. Once the three-dimensional structure of DNA became known, scientists tried to work out a theoretical basis on which DNA itself could serve as a direct template for the assembly of amino acids into a linear protein chain. It was imagined that different amino acids might somehow recognize and interact with groupings of three or four nucleotides in a row, lining up side by side on a portion of a DNA strand, on a gene. Once each amino acid formed a chemical bond with its neighbor, the result would be the protein specified by that gene. Because of the physical restrictions imposed by the Watson-Crick DNA model, such a straightforward idea could not be shown to work. How, then, could DNA direct the synthesis of new protein in a cell? This puzzle was finally solved when investigators turned their attention to the second form of nucleic acid present in all cells: *ribonucleic acid (RNA.)*

Like DNA, RNA is a linear polymer of nucleotides. Three of the four nucleotides in RNA correspond closely to the adenine, guanine, and cytosine found in DNA; the only difference is that the *deoxyribo*nucleotides lack a hydroxyl group found on the sugar component of *ribo*nucleotides. Moreover, the fourth nucleotide in RNA, uracil, takes the place of the thymine found in DNA. These slight differences in structure confer important chemical differences on RNA and DNA. Although two complementary RNA molecules can form double-stranded structures, they do not form a double helix as DNA does. Single-stranded RNA is made from DNA during the *transcription* process. The transcription of RNA from DNA proceeds in exactly the same way as the replication of DNA from DNA. The double-stranded structure opens up, and individual ribonucleotides assemble along one of the strands under the guidance of an enzyme called *RNA polymerase*. The ribonucleotides snap together as they are brought into place, forming a linear strand of RNA.

Unlike DNA, which is found almost exclusively in the nucleus, only a small portion of total cellular RNA is nuclear; most RNA is found in the cytoplasm.* The function of RNA was even more obscure at first than DNA. It was known that the majority of nonnuclear RNA was associated with dense cytoplasmic particles called *microsomes*. But since no one had the slightest idea what microsomes represented in terms of cellular function, the role of microsomal RNA was equally obscure.

In 1958 a key experiment by Elliot Volkin and Lazarus Astrachan showed that when phage infect a bacterium, there is an intense burst of new RNA synthesis. The newly synthesized RNA was fairly short lived, was found in association with the bacterial microsomes, and appeared to correlate well with new (phage) protein production. Even at its peak, this RNA represented only a small percentage of the total microsomal RNA. The most important point noted by Volkin and Astrachan, however, was that the nucleotide composition of the newly made RNA matched more closely the nucleotide composition of the *phage* DNA than the *bacterial* DNA. This raised the possibility that short-lived RNA might represent a "messenger" RNA made from the phage DNA, which then associated with bacterial microsomes for translation into protein.

It took awhile for this revolutionary idea — that RNA could act as an informational intermediate between DNA and protein — to sink in. But within a few years researchers working on protein synthesis talked of microsomes as the cellular site where protein synthesis took place under the direction of *messenger RNA* (*mRNA*). Messenger RNA, rather than DNA, was increasingly viewed as being the template for the actual assembly of amino acids into protein. It was thought likely that mRNA would

---

*The only other place DNA is found in a cell is in cytoplasmic structures called *mitochondria*, which are used to generate cellular energy. Mitochondria were formed in evolution when certain bacteria took up residence in larger cells, and used oxygen (which was just beginning to accumulate in the atmosphere) for energy generation. These bacteria eventually gave up their independence and degenerated into mitochondria, which still retain and use portions of the original bacterial DNA.

be copied from discrete regions of the DNA, from individual genes specifying individual proteins. The mRNA would thus be the functional equivalent of a xeroxed copy of a gene that is translated on the microsomes into a specific protein.

After Volkin and Astrachan's experiment, scientists increasingly turned their attention to the informational potential of mRNA. Most laboratories began by trying to isolate mRNA coding for specific proteins. There were several reasons for doing this, chief among which was that mRNA's proposed role in protein synthesis was still only a theory—it lacked experimental verification. But it was also clear that mRNA would be the key to solving the genetic code. By 1960 everyone believed that linear stretches of three or four nucleotides in mRNA would specify each of the twenty known amino acids. The only way to solve the code would be to determine the nucleotide sequence in an mRNA molecule, and compare it directly with the amino acid sequence of the protein it encoded.

The first task was to set up a system in which protein synthesis could be reliably and reproducibly measured, and in which a role for mRNA could be tested. Because it was not possible at the time to introduce mRNA into living cells where translation into protein could take place, researchers developed a system wherein bacteria or other cells could be broken open, and their contents transferred to a test tube. Under appropriate conditions, and if they were supplied with amino acids, a few salts, and an energy source, these "cell-free" systems were indeed able to use exogenously supplied mRNA to synthesize proteins.

Although the cell-free extracts could make protein in response to bulk RNA fractions from cells, attempts to isolate specific mRNAs coding for individual proteins proved fruitless for many years. Then, in 1961, two of the scientists pursuing this line of research had a remarkable piece of luck that allowed them not only to be the first to synthesize a protein from a piece of defined mRNA in a cell-free system, but provided them with the first "word" in the genetic code. Marshall Nirenberg and Johann Matthaei, working at the National Institutes of Health in Bethesda, Maryland, decided in the course of their experiments to use synthetic, rather than natural, mRNA as a template for protein synthesis. The ability to make linear RNA polymers had only recently been developed. They added a pure polymer of the nucleotide uridine ("poly U") to a bacterial cell-free system, and found that it induced the formation of a linear polymer made from only a single amino acid, phenylalanine. That meant that some number of uridines grouped together along a string of RNA instructed the system to incorporate the amino acid phenylalanine into a growing protein. The magic number would turn out to be three—the famous triplet unit or *codon* specifying each amino acid in the genetic code. The next codon to be identified, using a poly C template, was CCC, which specifies the amino acid proline.

Nirenberg and Matthaei's work was presented at a conference in Moscow in 1961. Nirenberg was completely unknown at the time, and not many of the leading scientists present at the meeting attended his talk. A few did, however, and the word spread rapidly that he was in the process of cracking the code. Francis Crick arranged for him to present his paper again in the final session, this time to a standing-room-only crowd.

The audience was stunned—but only momentarily. Everyone interested in the genetic code immediately rushed back to his or her laboratory and began constructing synthetic mRNAs of defined nucleotide sequence as a way of cracking the code. It was difficult work, and the competition was fierce. The importance of the quest itself was underscored by the title of Francis Crick's 1962 Nobel Prize address in Stockholm: "The Genetic Code." There was enormous excitement along the way, marvelous technical breakthroughs and compelling personal stories. Quite a few reputations were made (Nirenberg himself received a Nobel Prize in 1968 for his seminal contributions); more than one reputation was tarnished in the rush to be first. But by 1965, the work was essentially complete; the resulting code is shown in Figure 3-2. The code shown is for mRNA; the corresponding DNA code can be readily derived by substituting T for U and by making the appropriate nucleotide inversions (G for C; A for T; etc.). Although either code would be valid, molecular biologists routinely use the mRNA version shown here.

There are several important features to note about the genetic code. First, it is universal; the same code is used by every living organism on earth. There are few things nature has created that she doesn't eventually tinker with to some degree; the genetic code is one of them.* The reason for this rigid conservation is fairly straightforward; if the code were

---

*Mitochondrial DNA uses a very slightly modified version of the genetic code. Whether this represents a chemical "fossil" of the earliest form of the code, or degeneration due to specific needs within the cell, is unknown.

First Base of mRNA Codon	Second Base of mRNA Codon				Third Base of mRNA Codon
	U	C	A	G	
U	UUU Phe UUC Phe UUA Leu UUG Leu	UCU Ser UCC Ser UCA Ser UCG Ser	UAU Tyr UAC Tyr UAA stop UAG stop	UGU Cys UGC Cys UGA stop UGG Trp	U C A G
C	CUU Leu CUC Leu CUA Leu CUG Leu	CCU Pro CCC Pro CCA Pro CCG Pro	CAU His CAC His CAA Gln CAG Gln	CGU Arg CGC Arg CGA Arg CGG Arg	U C A G
A	AUU Ile AUC Ile AUA Ile AUG start	ACU Thr ACC Thr ACA Thr ACG Thr	AAU Asn AAC Asn AAA Lys AAG Lys	AGU Ser AGC Ser AGA Arg AGG Arg	U C A G
G	GUU Val GUC Val GUA Val GUG Val	GCU Ala GCC Ala GCA Ala GCG Ala	GAU Asp GAC Asp GAA Gln GAG Gln	GGU Gly GGC Gly GGA Gly GGG Gly	U C A G

Figure 3-2. The genetic code. The possible triplets that can be formed by combination of the four different RNA nucleotides are displayed in this standard table. The triplets are displayed in upper case letters, followed by the three-letter abbreviation of the corresponding amino acid the triplet encodes.

changed for even one amino acid, it would mean that that amino acid would have to change in every single protein in a living cell, without altering the structural and functional integrity of each of those proteins. It is impossible to imagine how this might be done.

The second thing about the code is that it is redundant (or, as molecular biologists like to put it, *degenerate*). Four nucleotides randomly grouped into triplets can make sixty-four different "words." Thus, most of the twenty different amino acids are encoded by more than one codon; only the amino acid tryptophan (*trp)* is specified by a single codon. Some amino acids (e.g., *leu*cine, *ser*ine and *arg*ine) are encoded by six different triplets. Finally, some of the possible codons are not used for words at all; they are used for punctuation. AUG, for example, is used to mark the beginning of a "sentence" — the beginning of an encoded amino acid sequence defining a protein. That answers an important question noted by biologists even before the code was solved: Given that a linear sequence of nucleotides would have to be read off three or four at a time, how

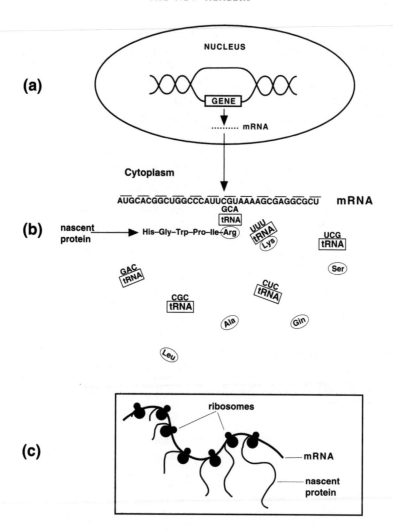

Figure 3-3. Transcription and translation.

would the proper message be read? Shifting one nucleotide to the right or left in reading a message would lead to the production of an entirely different message! And how would the cell know when a message has ended? That is where UAA, UAG, or UGA come in — they serve as a periods.

The way in which DNA and RNA work together in the production of proteins is shown in Figure 3-3. Gene expression begins when the DNA strands partially unwind in the vicinity of a gene (Figure 3-3a), allowing the transcriptional machinery access to the control sites just upstream (5') of the gene. The gene is transcribed into an mRNA copy which is processed and exported to the cytoplasm for translation (Figure 3-3b). Amino acids are brought to the mRNA by special tRNA transporters. The tRNAs have an "anti-sense" codon triplet that allows them to bind to the mRNA. Each such codon-specific tRNA also has a separate binding site for the amino acid represented by the codon it recognizes. As successive tRNAs bring their amino acids to the nascent protein chain, special enzymes form a peptide bond between the new amino acid and the growing protein chain. This happens through the mediation of dumbbell-shaped ribosomes (Figure 3-3c; note change in scale!). Ribosomes attach to mRNA at one end (the left hand as shown here) and move down the mRNA one codon at a time. At each codon the ribosome stops until the proper tRNA has brought the requisite amino acid. As soon as the peptide bond forms between the new amino acid and the nascent chain, the ribosome moves over by exactly one codon position, dragging the growing protein chain with it. When a ribosome has moved along far enough, another ribosome attaches attach at the free end; a dozen or so ribosomes may be moving down an mRNA molecule at any give point during translation. The ribosomes furthest along on the mRNA will have the longest newly forming proteins dangling from them. When a ribosome reaches a stop codon, the ribosome falls apart, releasing the completed protein molecule for use by the cell.

The transcription and translation processes involved in reading the genes that are a natural part of a cell's own DNA are exactly the same processes used to "read" foreign genes introduced into a cell in the treatment known as gene therapy. The detailed knowledge gained over the past four decades about how these processes work in a living cell is the foundation upon which molecular medicine is built.

Genetic Mutations

We now know what genes are: specific sequences of nucleotides arranged along a DNA strand, with start and stop signals, and written in a triplet-based code that we can read. We know what genes do: they dictate the sequences of amino acids that make up the proteins in our bodies. Genetic diseases (diseases caused by defective genes) arise when these genes accumulate *mutations*, and an understanding of exactly what mutations are is important in understanding what gene therapy is intended to correct.

Genetic mutations refer to any alteration in the inherited nucleic acid sequence of the genotype of an organism. Traditionally, geneticists defined mutations operationally; i.e., only in terms of those genotypic changes resulting in some change in the resulting phenotype. However, as scientists developed the ability to measure changes directly in DNA itself, the definition of mutation has expanded to include any alteration in DNA, whether or not the alteration occurs in a gene, and whether or not the altered gene results in an altered phenotype.

Mutations may be caused in several ways. Radiation from an X-ray machine or a gamma-ray source can cause mutations, as can the radiation from nuclear disintegrations. Certain chemicals we refer to as *mutagens* can cause alterations in the nucleic acid sequences of genes. Probably the most common source of mutations are those arising from mistakes made during the DNA replication. DNA replication is very carefully regulated, with many "proofreading" safeguards built in to detect mistakes, but the process is not perfect. Each time a human cell divides, it must reassemble six *billion* nucleotides into a complete chromosomal set. The mistake rate may be as high as one nucleotide in ten thousand, which would mean as many as a half million or more mistakes. The cell is equipped with repair mechanisms that allow it to detect mutations from any source, and the vast majority of mistakes are corrected before they cause any harm; Occasionally, however, one will slip through. Should this happen in the germ cells (the sperm or ova), the mutation will be passed on to the next generation, where it will affect every cell in the body of the offspring including its germ cells. In this fashion, a single germ-cell mutation may be passed on to innumerable future generations. If a mutation occurs in a cell other than a germ cell (i.e., in a somatic cell), the effect of the mutation will be limited to that cell, or, at most, to its immediate descendants within the body. The mutation in this case disappears with the organism at death, and will not be passed on to future generations.

Mutations can be of several types. Those involving only a single nucleotide change are referred to as *point mutations*, and may include exchanges of one nucleotide for another, or the additon or deletion of a single nucleotide (Figure 3-4). Exchanging one nucleic acid for another can have several effects. It may generate a stop codon, which will disrupt the translation process (Figure 3-4c). It could also change a stop codon to an amino acid codon, and the translation process may proceed beyond the normal end of the protein. Changing a nucleotide in a codon will in

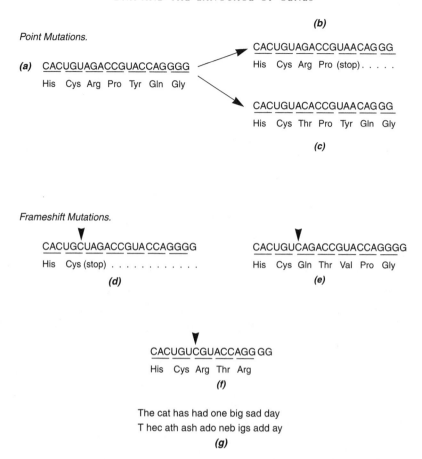

Point Mutations.

(b)

(a) CACUGUAGACCGUACCAGGGG

His Cys Arg Pro Tyr Gln Gly

CACUGUAGACCGUAACAGGG

His Cys Arg Pro (stop). . . . .

CACUGUACACCGUAACAGGG

His Cys Thr Pro Tyr Gln Gly

(c)

Frameshift Mutations.

CACUGCUAGACCGUACCAGGGG

His Cys (stop) . . . .

(d)

CACUGUCAGACCGUACCAGGGG

His Cys Gln Thr Val Pro Gly

(e)

CACUGUCGUACCAGGGG

His Cys Arg Thr Arg

(f)

The cat has had one big sad day

T hec ath ash ado neb igs add ay

(g)

Figure 3-4. DNA alterations (mutations) affecting protein structure. The alterations shown here are seen at the mRNA level to conform with the genetic code given in Figure 3-2. In (d), a "C" (arrow) has been inserted after the fifth nucleotide from the left in (a). This shifts the reading frame one nucleotide to the right, generating a premature stop codon. In (e), a "C" has been inserted after the sixth nucleotide in (a), shifting the reading frame one nucleotide to the right which results in a protein that the cell will not be able to use. In (f), a block of four nucleotides occurring just after the fifth nucleotide from the right in (a) has been deleted, again causing a frameshift and production of a nonsense protein.

most, but not all, cases change the amino acid specified by the codon (Figure 3-4b). For example, substitution of a C for the G in the codon AGA, which specifies the amino acid arginine, results in ACA, which specifies threonine. There are many examples where a single nucleotide alteration, and the consequent change in a single amino acid, results in disease or even death. Depending on the new amino acid's importance for the protein's function, it is possible that the change may have no impact; on very rare occasions, the new amino acid might even work better. But after hundreds of millions of years of evolution, the amino acid sequence of most proteins is fairly optimal; most amino acid changes are harmful or, at best, neutral. Protein function is very sensitive to the way a protein folds itself in three-dimensional space, and this is determined by the protein's amino acid sequence. Many mutations, and the resulting amino acid substitutions, strongly affect protein folding. If the protein is an enzyme, certain amino acids in the protein will also be involved with specific enzymatic function. Mutations in these amino acids are almost always harmful.

The addition or deletion of a single nucleotide is always lethal for the affected gene, because this causes what is known as a *frameshift mutation*. As shown in Figure 3-4d, adding or deleting a nucleic acid puts the nucleic acids *downstream* of the change into a different reading frame, and all amino acids after that point will be completely different than what was originally specified by the inherited gene. The resulting protein will be completely nonsensical, and will likely be destroyed by the cell in which it is made. The way in which a frameshift can generate nonsense is shown in (Figure 3-4g), using an English sentence based on three-letter words.

Frameshifts can also be caused by the deletion or insertion of larger blocks of nucleic acids. These blocks may or may not alter the reading frame of the gene, leading to nonsense sequences or early termination, depending on whether or not they occur as multiples of three nucleic acids, and whether they are in or out of frame. The predominant mutation in the CF gene, as we will see in Chapter 7, involves the deletion of three nucleotides forming an in-frame triplet encoding phenylalanine. Another example of this type of mutation is seen in Huntington's disease, a uniformly fatal, hereditary neurodegenerative disorder that will be discussed in more detail later. Huntington's disease is caused by the insertion of multiple in-frame repeats of the codon CAG (which encodes glutamine) into a gene called *IT15*. The Huntington's protein thus has an abnormally long stretch of polyglutamine at one end. The function of this protein is not known at present, but the mutational effect is dominant; inheritance of a single mutated allele of the Huntington's gene is sufficient to cause this invariably fatal disease.

The purpose of gene therapy in most cases is to correct the consequences of having inherited mutant copies of a given gene. The mutation to be corrected did not arise in the individual with the genetic disease; it arose in one or more of his or her forebears. To correct the problem caused by this hereditary accident, it is necessary to identify the gene involved, to isolate normal copies of the gene, and to deliver them to cells of the affected individual. We will see how this is done in Chapter 5. But, before we do that, let us take a look at another genetic disease, one that was the target for the very first clinical trial of human gene therapy: severe combined immune deficiency, or SCID.

4

Severe Combined Immunodeficiency Disease

Severe combined immunodeficiency disease (SCID) is truly as bad as it sounds. As with cystic fibrosis, SCID is an inherited disease involving mutations of a single gene in an afflicted child. But unlike CF, where there is only one gene in the entire human population responsible for the disease, SCID can be caused by mutations in any one of a number of different genes affecting largely the T cell arm of the immune response. In CF, defects in the single gene responsible, the chloride ion transporter (CFTR), affect a wide range of cells and tissues in the body, resulting in a spectrum of seemingly unrelated disorders. In SCID, defects in several quite distinct genes can cripple a single type of white blood cell (the T lymphocyte or *T cell*), causing a single, highly focussed medical problem: susceptibility to infectious disease. When untreated, SCID is uniformly lethal within the first year or two of life. Fortunately, SCID is a relatively rare genetic disorder; only about forty "SCID kids" are born each year in the U.S. Unfortunately, it is extremely difficult to treat, and the majority of affected children still die of the disease.

To understand why SCID is such a deadly disease, we need to take a brief look at how the immune system is organized. The immune system protects us against infectious disease, caused by microbial life forms that manage to break through the body's first lines of defense, such as skin or mucus-coated epithelial surfaces. Human beings evolved in a world teeming with disease-causing (pathogenic) microbes. These microbes — principally bacteria, viruses, funguses, and a few parasites thrown in for good measure — inhabit every possible niche on the planet. They are found at the bottom of the sea, under enormous bathymetric pressure, sometimes at the rim of boiling-hot sulfur vents; they also do just fine in frozen arctic tundra. So it should come as no surprise that they find a warm, dark, moist human body an ideal place to live and reproduce.

To deal with the challenge to our well-being posed by these microbial pathogens, humans (along with other vertebrate animals) evolved an incredibly powerful and effective immune system. The elements of the immune system we need to be familiar with in order to understand what goes wrong in SCID are shown in Figure 4-1. The immune system mounts several kinds of attacks on foreign invaders. One arm of the immune system is based on a type of white blood cell called a *B cell*. B cells make proteins called *antibodies*, which they release into the bloodstream in response to invasion by anything foreign, such as a bacterium. The antibody binds to the bacterium, tagging it for disposal. A second type of white blood cell, called a *macrophage*, is able to detect objects that have been tagged by antibody, and will engulf them and destroy them. But in order to develop properly and to make antibody, B cells need help from yet another white blood cell, called a *T Helper cell*. Helper T cells provide chemical signals needed by B cells to enter into antibody production. Helper T cells display a special surface molecule called CD4 , and thus are also called CD4 T cells. These are the T cells infected and killed by the AIDS virus, HIV. Without T cell help, B cells are greatly compromised in their ability to respond to foreign invasion, and the antibody arm of the immune response is drastically reduced.

Another type of T cell, called a killer T cell or a CD8 T cell, carries out the second major form of immune defense against pathogens. CD8 T cells have the special property of being able to detect cells in the body that have been invaded by intracellular pathogens such as viruses. (Bacteria live mostly outside of cells, in the blood or other body fluids. Viruses, and a few bacteria, live inside our cells where antibody cannot

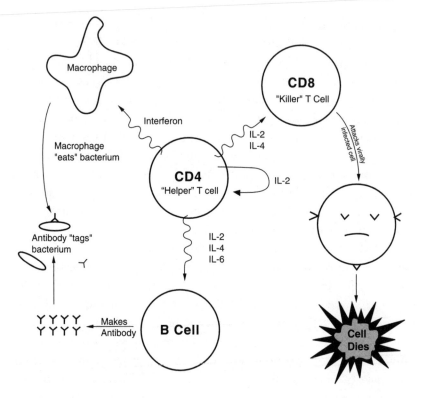

Figure 4-1. Cellular interactions in the immune system.

reach them). When a CD8 T cell determines that a cell has been sub-verted by an invader, it attacks and destroys that cell, to deprive the pathogen within of a place to live and reproduce. CD8 T cells also need help from CD4 T cells as they develop in the body.

Notice that both types of immune response—antibody production as well as direct killing of infected cells—are dependent on helper T cells. CD4 T cells are often referred to as the master conductors of the immunological orchestra, and this is true to a considerable degree. Both types of T cells produce a number of chemical signals, called *interleukins*. These small protein molecules are used by other cells of the immune sys-tem to carry out their specific functions. Some of the interleukins stim-ulate activity in other immune cells; other interleukins are involved in turning down the action slightly when the immune system appears to be overreacting.

It is clear that if T cells are compromised, the immune system is effectively shut down. SCID children are born without T cell function and, thus, for all practical purposes, without an immune system. There are other cells in the immune system, such as *neutrophils* and the macrophages themselves, that can offer some degree of protection against bacterial infection. However, humans have come to rely almost entirely on T cells for protection against many viruses. Although elements of the immune system other than T and B cells are certainly important and useful, the fact remains that, if untreated, SCID is uniformly fatal. This is what happens in the final stages of AIDS, when a virus (HIV, the human immunodeficiency virus) infects and destroys the patient's CD4 T cells. Like all infants, SCID children are born with antibodies passed through the mother's placenta, and additional protection may come from the antibodies in breast milk. But this protection wears off within the first year of life, and antibodies are, at best, only partially effective against viruses and funguses.

Like AIDS patients, SCID children are particularly susceptible to *opportunistic infections*. These infections arise from pathogens already inside the body as a result of a previous infection that was controlled but not completely cleared by the immune system. In most cases the initial infection is controlled quickly enough so that the individual involved may not even have experienced any symptoms of disease. But a small number of the pathogenic microbes may somehow manage to hide in tissues or cells where they are relatively safe from the immune system. Normally, whenever they try to come out of these tissues or cells, they are rapidly detected and eliminated. Many of us carry these pathogens all our lives, but the immune system keeps them in check and we rarely experience the disease they represent. It is only when the immune system is compromised by some other problem, such as SCID or AIDS, that these pathogens are given the opportunity to roam freely in the body and wreak havoc unopposed.

The opportunistic infections seen in SCID patients can be very deadly. The fungus *Pneumocystis carinii* is found in many healthy people, largely in the lungs. In people with compromised immune systems, *P. carinii* causes a particularly severe form of pneumonia that is difficult to treat. It can be managed to some degree by drugs like *pentamidine*, which can be sprayed directly into the lungs, but it remains one of the most life-threatening diseases in SCID children. SCID patients also suffer from a number of opportunistic viruses that are relatively harmless to the population as a whole, such as *cytomegalovirus* (*CMV*), which is a member of the herpes family of virus. Approximately half of the U.S. population is infected with CMV, but people with healthy immune symptoms are rarely symptomatic. In SCID patients CMV causes a wide range of serious health problems, including a type of pneumonia as well as ulcers, brain and liver damage, and blindness. Type I and II herpes viruses, relatively harmless in most people, can be a very serious problem for SCID patients.

For infants with SCID, bacterial and fungal infections can be controlled to some extent by antibiotic treatment, but little can be done to manage viral infections, which are a common cause of death. In the past the only hope for long-term survival for many forms of SCID has been a bone marrow transplant, preferably from a tissue-matched sibling. Both T and B cells arise from hematopoeitic (blood-forming) *stem cells* in the bone marrow, and bone marrow from a SCID-free donor has at least the potential to correct the underlying defect. But even then the outlook is poor; only about a third of those receiving a transplant survive beyond a few years.

David in his Bubble: X-linked SCID

The nation became suddenly aware of SCID through the dramatic and ultimately tragic case of a young boy named David, who was born in Texas in 1971. (David's full name was never made public.) The type of SCID young David suffered from was caused by defects in a single gene that, like the gene in CF, is inherited in standard Mendelian fashion. This particular gene is located on the X chromosome, and so the disease is referred to as *X-linked SCID*, or simply *X-SCID*. Human males, being XY, have a single X chromosome. Thus unlike the situation in CF, where a child must inherit a defective gene from each parent, young X-SCID males develop their disease through inheritance of a single defective gene on the X chromosome from their mothers. (Normally only females are carriers of this disease, since males do not usually live long enough to reproduce.) Thus half of the male offspring of a carrier mother will be born with SCID; half the daughters will, like their mothers, be heterozygous carriers. Roughly half of all SCID cases involve X-SCID.

David's parents had lost an infant son to X-SCID less than two years earlier, so the possibility of a second male child with SCID was known well in advance. The first child developed severe infections at five months of age, and died at seven months. Midterm amniocentesis had indicated that David would in fact be male, although at the time it was not possible to determine whether he carried a defective gene. At any rate, the family did not consider abortion to be an option. David was delivered by caesarian section (to prevent contact with the microbes that are a normal part of vaginal birth) and was immediately transferred to a sterile incubator until his immune status could be determined. Within a short time it was learned that he, too, had inherited the defective gene causing SCID.

Since the sterile environment protected him from disease-causing microbes, and since he had not yet picked up his own opportunistic pathogens, young David quickly became the longest living untreated SCID patient. The idea behind this approach to managing a child with SCID was the hope that if he could be kept alive long enough in the absence of disease, his immune system might somehow "kick in" and allow him to defend himself; this was not an unreasonable hope at the time. Over the next several months he was tested for signs of T cell responsiveness, but the cells never became functional. When he began to crawl and eventually to stand, he was moved into a sterile tent that allowed some freedom of movement, consistent with the need to protect him from environmental pathogens. As he continued to grow, the tent eventually became "the Bubble," an ingenious complex of interconnecting plastic tubes that allowed him to move around and explore, in an environment full of variously shaped and colored objects to stimulate his senses of vision and touch. It was constructed in such a way as to allow maximal interactivity with family and playmates on the outside. NASA even built a small space suit for him so he could gain some impression of independent movement in the outside world; he outgrew it within a year. A sterile transporter was developed so that he could be taken home, and learn what it means to be part of a nuclear family. He was given a good education at home in his bubble; his nurses and tutors found him to be a bright, somewhat mischievous youngster, not obviously distinguishable from other boys his age.

But his immune system never developed. As David continued to grow, it became clear that something had to be done. He was healthy and vigorous, and very clever: What if he tried to break out of his bubble? And at twelve years of age he was showing the first signs of normal sexual maturation. No one had thought this far ahead; his medical team found themselves in an enormous and unprecedented ethical dilemma, with no guidelines for how to proceed. How long could someone survive in a sterile bubble? In the beginning doctors were worried that he would not survive long, and now they had to deal with the possibility that he might; there was nothing to suggest that his life would be foreshortened by his disease. What would be the psychological and spiritual state of a person living out an entire life span under these conditions?

Finally, it was decided to give David a bone marrow transplant, with his fifteen-year-old sister Katherine as the donor. David and his sister were not particularly tissue compatible, which is one reason a transplant with her marrow had not been attempted earlier. The chance for success with poorly matched marrow was less than fifty-fifty at the time. In late 1983, when David received his sister's marrow, there were only about two dozen SCID children in the world that had been successfully transplanted, and nearly all of these were with closely matched donor marrow. Nevertheless, it was decided to take the risk. David was taken to a sterile operating room and infused with his sister's bone marrow. He was kept briefly in a sterile postoperative recovery room, and then returned to his bubble.

Everything seemed to go well at first. But a few weeks later he developed symptoms that seemed possibly related to one of the principal dangers of bone marrow transplantation: GVH ("graft-vs.-host") disease. GVH disease arises when mature T cells in the donor bone marrow settle into the recipient's body and begin to regard it as a huge organ transplant. The graft in this case begins to reject the host. Appropriate steps were taken immediately to control GVH, but to no avail. There were also puzzling signs of a viral infection. David's condition grew rapidly worse; he finally died on the one hundred and twenty-fourth day post-transplant. He was twelve years old.

It turned out that David did not die from complications of GVH disease; in fact hematopoietic stem cells from his sister's bone marrow had failed completely to implant and function in his body. He died of congestive heart failure secondary to a B cell lymphoma. His sister, like much of the population, carried an opportunistic pathogen called the Epstein-Barr virus (EBV) in her blood cells. EBV is normally kept under control by the body's immune system; when it occasionally breaks out, it may cause a flu-like state known as *mononucleosis*. In patients with a compromised immune system, however, it can progress into a deadly form of cancer, called B cell lymphoma. Bone marrow is always contaminated with blood that seeps in during its removal from bone cavities. Once inside David's own system, EBV apparently escaped from his sister's blood cells and infected his own B cells, some of which eventually became cancerous.

Just before David died, some of his T cells were harvested and frozen away for future study. In 1993, scientists working with DNA isolated from his cells, among others, were able to pinpoint the defective gene that caused his form of SCID. The gene encodes a protein found on the surface of T cells that allows them to receive a crucial chemical growth signal (see IL-2; see Figure 4-1) from the environment. This growth factor receptor is absolutely crucial to the normal development of T cells in the body; without it their growth is halted at a very early stage, and they die. Because of the key role played by T cells in immune responsiveness, the patient is left with only the most rudimentary immune defenses. The IL-2 receptor gene has now been isolated and "cloned" by means we will discuss in the next chapter, and should be ready for gene therapy trials in the very near future.

ADA SCID

There is another form of SCID, equally as deadly as the X-SCID that afflicted David, called ADA-SCID. ADA-SCID accounts for roughly a quarter of all SCID cases seen clinically in the United States. Although ADA-SCID results in exactly the same disease symptoms that David experienced, the underlying genetic defect is completely different. ADA-SCID is caused by a mutation in the gene that codes for an enzyme called *adenosine deaminase (ADA)*, which is involved in the metabolism of one of the nucleotide precursors used to assemble DNA. The gene for ADA is not X-linked, but rather is found on one of the other chromosome pairs. As in CF, development of ADA-SCID requires the inheritance of *two* defective gene copies, one from each parent. This in turn requires that both parents are heterozygous (carriers) for the ADA gene: each has one good copy, and one bad copy. As predicted by standard Mendelian genetics, one in four offspring (regardless of sex) will inherit two defective gene copies, and develop ADA-SCID. ADA is an enzyme used in all cells of the body, and someone born with two defective copies of the ADA gene has no ADA whatsoever. This leads to a buildup of a chemical called *deoxyadenosine*. This is not a problem for most cells, but T cells convert the deoxyadenosine into another chemical which is exceedingly toxic, and

63

the cells die. Children born with no ADA thus lose all their T cells, and suffer exactly the same set of consequences as children with X-SCID.

Just a short time before gene therapy trials for ADA-SCID were proposed, it became possible to give patients the ADA enzyme itself, in a form known as PEG-ADA (which is polyethylene glycol attached to the ADA molecule). Enough of it may get into the developing T cells to rescue them before they die. But in the case of a four-year-old girl named Ashanti DeSilva, even this form of therapy had not worked. By September of 1990, the T cells in her blood had fallen to a level ordinarily seen only in patients in the terminal stages of AIDS. As in David's case, there was no well-matched sibling to act as a donor, so a bone-marrow transplant was considered too risky. Her family and doctors were running out of options. But this young lady would be offered an option never before given any human being: she would be invited to become the very first human gene therapy patient.

Fittingly, this foray into the medicine of the future would take place at the National Institutes of Health, literally yards from where Marshall Nirenberg and Johann Matthaei had cracked the genetic code thirty years before, in a project headed by one of Nirenberg's disciples. That very same code had been used to work out the sequence of the human ADA gene in the 1980s; now that gene would be the first piece of genetically engineered DNA to enter a human body for the express purpose of correcting an inborn genetic defect. Three physician-scientists at NIH — Dr. W. French Anderson, Dr. Michael Blaese, and Dr. Kenneth Culver — had just received clearance from government oversight committees to use the ADA gene for treating human disease. They turned to young Ashanti as their first patient.

In this first gene therapy trial, it was decided to introduce a normal, healthy copy of the ADA gene directly into her T cells. A few of her scarce T cells were withdrawn from her blood and placed into culture dishes under conditions that would cause them to grow and expand, and they were exposed during this growth period to literally billions of copies of the healthy gene. No attempt was made to "repair" her faulty gene copies, nor were they removed from her DNA. The fact that heterozygotes (her parents, for example) carrying one bad copy of the gene do not have the disease tells us that the presence of a bad ADA gene does not compromise the function of a good ADA gene. It also tells us that a single good copy is enough to support normal cell function. After a week and a half of growth and exposure to the ADA gene, her modified T cells were placed back into her bloodstream through a simple intravenous drip.

And so one of the monumental moments of medical science passed very quietly. No heroic surgery, no lights or cameras. Just a cloudy suspension of cells dripping for a half hour or so into the forearm of a rather shy four-year-old girl. After the infusion, Ashi, as she was called, was monitored closely for any signs of an adverse reaction; there were none. Her temperature, pulse, and blood pressure remained normal. As a precaution, she has been kept on PEG-ADA throughout the trial. After another infusion a month later, the level of healthy T cells in her blood began to climb. Some of these cells were taken back to the lab and examined for their expression of the healthy ADA. The new gene had indeed found its way into the DNA of her T cells, and was rescuing them—and her—from death.

Most importantly, little Ashi began to show signs of being able to make antibodies, proving that the repaired T cells were able to carry out one of their key functions: helping B cells. She also showed signs of having acquired T-cell functions associated with the ability to kill virally infected cells. Within less than a year, her T cell count was 1,250—well within the normal range for healthy humans. Her parents reported an overall improvement in her health and vitality. A second young girl with ADA-SCID was treated by exactly the same procedure just a few months after Ashi. Both of these young ladies now have vastly improved T cell function, and more vigorous and healthy immune systems generally. They attend school and are very active in, among other things, the national March of Dimes campaign to raise funds for childhood diseases. To date a total of eleven children have been treated for ADA-SCID by gene therapy.

And so the medical revolution that may change the face of medicine in the twenty-first century was actually born in the final decade of the twentieth. The first use of antibodies in the treatment of infectious disease happened at almost the same point in the nineteenth century. It is impossible to say now whether gene therapy will have as profound an effect on human health as immune therapy did one hundred years ago. But it certainly has that potential.

ADA-SCID clinical trials were begun in 1990, and CF trials were started in 1994; those for X-linked SCID are about to get underway. Over two hundred clinical trials for a number of additional genetic disorders, as well as cancer and AIDS, have cleared federal regulatory agencies; most are already underway. The scientific and medical communities are watching these trials closely, and so will the public. There will likely be close media coverage of the progress of patients involved in one or another of these medical dramas. The challenges posed by these first trials — scientific, medical, and ethical — are fairly typical of what we will see in the treatment of medical problems as wide-ranging as vascular disease, hemophilia, arthritis, and liver disorders. In the next few chapters we will examine the proposed gene therapy treatments for CF and SCID, and the scientific strategies on which they are based, in more detail. We are coming close to the type of understanding all of us will need in the very near future, if we are to play a fully informed role in the care of our own health and that of our families.

5

The Isolation, Cloning, and Transfer of Human Genes

When Walter Sutton set forth, in 1903, his notion that Mendel's "factors of heredity" (later called genes) must be physically discrete entities arranged along chromosomes, he also noted that the total number of such factors necessary to specify an entire living organism — plant or animal — would surely far exceed the number of chromosomes found in individual cells of that organism. For those who accepted Sutton's point of view, it became of interest to see whether or not and to what extent specific genes are in fact associated with specific chromosomes, and perhaps even specific locations (*loci*) on specific chromosomes.

The answer was not long in coming. Thomas Hunt Morgan, whose work with the common fruit fly *Drosophila melanogaster* would lay the foundation for classical genetics for the next fifty years, showed in 1910 that the gene for white eye color in *Drosophila* (the normal color is red) was always associated with the X chromosome. As in humans, *Drosophila* males are XY, and the female is XX. Within three years Alfred Sturtevant, an undergraduate student working in Morgan's laboratory, described five more genes associated with the X chromosome in fruit flies, and moreover established that these six genes always occur in the same order on all *Drosophila* X chromosomes. This provided the very first gene map. (The production of such maps for the estimated 100,000 or so human genes is one of the goals of the Human Genome Project, which we will discuss in Chapter 12.) The way Sturtevant made his X chromosome map is shown in Figure 5-1. It is important to have some appreciation of his approach, because it is at the very heart of classical gene mapping. The method he developed over eighty years ago is still in use today.

First of all, how did Sturtevant know his six genes were associated with the X chromosome, and not one of the other three chromosomes making up the *Drosophila* genome? It must be remembered that in the early days of gene study, the existence of a gene was inferred only by the existence of mutations affecting the phenotype. Mutations with a clear phenotype are very useful in following the inheritance of genes. In a heterozygote, most mutations are "invisible" because they are recessive; the presence of one good gene compensates for the mutated form of the gene. But in males, genes uniquely associated with the X chromosome are present in only one copy per cell because there is only one X chromosome per cell; if that gene copy is mutant, then the cell (and the organism) will express the mutant phenotype. When a male with a mutant X-associated gene mates with a normal female, *all* of the daughters (XX) will be heterozygous for (i.e., will be carriers of) the mutation for that gene; none of the male offspring (XY) will have the gene. If the mutant gene were on any other chromosome, only half of the daughters would receive it, as would half of the sons. It is this unique inheritance pattern that makes it fairly easy to establish association of a gene with the X chromosome. Human disorders such as color blindness and hemophilia were associated on this basis with the X chromosome long before the human X chromosome was seen in a microscope.

Sturtevant had in hand a total of six X-linked genes. But how could he establish the order of the genes on the chromosome? This came about as a result of trying to understand the phenomenon of *crossing over* first detected by Morgan. In genetic parlance, the six genes on the X chromosome are considered to be "linked"; that is, during reproduction, they should all travel together because they are on the same chromosome. But

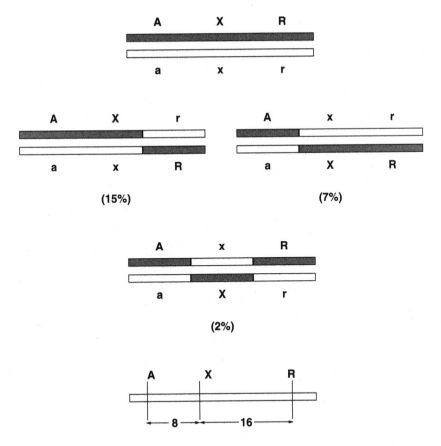

Figure 5-1. Determining gene order from crossing-over events. A, R and X are the dominant alleles of three genes determined to be linked on the same chromosome. a, r and x are the corresponding recessive alleles. Crossing over between X and R occurs in 15 percent of matings; between A and X in 7 percent of matings. This tells us about the relative distances between A and X, and X and R, but not about their absolute order. The crucial piece of evidence comes from the double crossing-over events involving these three loci, which occur in two percent of matings. The results for the crossing-over events shown could only be explained if X lies between A and R. These data allow the construction of a genetic map as shown at the bottom of the figure, where the numbers indicated are relative map units (called *Morgans*, after their originator.)

a detailed analysis of large numbers of breedings suggested that this is not always so. During the process of meiosis, when the two sets of chromosomes in every cell are reduced to one set in the germ cells, the two copies of each chromosome pair join together briefly, and occasionally exchange chromosomal segments with one another (see Figure 1-4). This provides yet another way of "scrambling" genetic information in order to create the new genetic combinations that natural selection acts upon. The genes per se remain associated with the same chromosome, but maternal and paternal alleles of the genes may reassociate along the chromosome, such that in the recombinant chromosome passed on to the next generation there is a mixing together of completely new and unique combination of alleles.

Sturtevant and Morgan reasoned that the frequency with which crossing over occurs between two genes on the same chromosome must be proportional to the physical distance between them. Assuming crossing over to be a random event, it should be more likely to occur between two genes at opposite ends of a chromosome than two genes immediately adjacent to one another. To a first approximation this is true, and the frequency of crossing over between the various possible paired combinations of Sturtevant's six genes was used to establish the relative distance between them, and to establish their relative order on the chromosome. Thus began the science (some would say the art) of chromosome mapping.

Assigning a given gene to the X chromosome is fairly straightforward because of the unique inheritance and expression patterns of such genes. But how can one make assignments of genes to other chromosomes? For many years, this was not possible. Genes could be sorted into "linkage groups" based on the fact that during breeding they tended to be passed on as discrete packages, presumably as discrete chromosomes. But which linkage groups represented which chromosomes was not at all clear. An important advance was made with the 1960s development of a technique called *somatic cell genetics*. The basic idea behind this technique is rather simple. When cells from two different species are fused together, the nuclei also fuse, and the chromosomes mix together in a single large nucleus. The hybrid cell functions relatively normally, and the genes of both sets of proteins are able to direct synthesis of proteins. However, over time chromosomes tend to be lost during cell division. In the case of human cells fused with rodent cells, it is almost always the human chromosomes that are lost. Eventually a cell line can be derived that has a normal complement of rodent chromosomes and a single human chromosome. By determining which human proteins are made by this cell, the gene for those proteins (and by inference all of the other genes in the same linkage group) can be assigned to the remaining chromosome.

Cutting DNA Down to Size

Once the chemical nature of DNA became known and the genetic code had been deciphered, determining the precise nucleotide sequence and overall organization of individual genes strung along the chromosomes became one of the most hotly pursued topics in all of biology. Clearly genes would be written in the basic genetic code; translation of this code would allow the determination of the amino acid sequence of the proteins encoded by the genes, which in turn could give some insight into their function. As more and more protein sequences became available for comparison with each other, it was noted that proteins sharing certain functions (enzymatic activity, insertion into a cell membrane, structural proteins) also shared certain amino acid sequences and motifs. For example, the amino acid sequence of the CFTR gene, when it was finally determined, was a major clue to the probable function of the defective protein in cystic fibrosis.

The ability to sequence DNA greatly facilitated the accumulation of protein sequence information, because nucleotide sequencing is at least ten times more rapid than amino acid sequencing. Getting the amino acid sequence of a protein directly is an unusually laborious process, starting at one end of the protein, chemically cleaving the amino acids one by one, and putting each of them through an analyzer that can recognize individual amino acids. At a scientific meeting in the late 1970s, the complete amino acid sequence of an important human protein, which had taken five years to work out in its entirety, was proudly presented by a distinguished senior scientist to an enthralled audience. About three talks farther into the program, a young "gene jock," as they were starting to be called, got up and made a statement to the effect that he had sequenced the gene for the same protein the month before, and he pointed out that the previous speaker had made a mistake: the amino acid at position 322 was a phenylalanine, not a leucine. It was immediately obvious to everyone in the room—painfully obvious to some, happily obvious to others —that the days of direct chemical sequencing of entire proteins was over. The complete sequence of a gene, and thus of the corresponding protein, can now often be obtained in a matter of weeks.

In addition to being read by the cell to determine protein sequence, we can infer that genes must also contain information that regulates their expression. We have known for many years that all genes are physically present in all cells; yet not every gene is expressed (transcribed and trans-lated) in every cell. For example, the gene for insulin is expressed in the pancreatic β-cells that make and secrete insulin, but not in other cells. The gene for melanin is "turned on" in skin cells, but not in blood cells. Moreover, even in cells where a gene is functioning, it often doesn't func-tion all the time, but only in response to specific signals. Pancreatic β-cells only turn on the insulin gene when intracellular stores of insulin are depleted in response to high blood-sugar levels outside the cell. How is selective gene expression regulated? It seemed likely from the beginning that genes would contain not only information dictating the sequence of a protein, but also nearby stretches of DNA through which regulatory signals could be received. What would these stretches look like? Where would they be located? In what kind of code would they be written?

The answer to these and other questions about gene structure and function could only be answered by isolating and studying individual genes. That meant, first of all, breaking down chromosomal DNA into sizes that could be worked with in the laboratory. For many years this was a major barrier to the isolation of individual genes for study. The human genome is enormous. It is made up of over three billion nucleotide pairs.* If we were to write out the nucleotide sequence of the entire human genome, it would require a million and a half pages, or about 6,000 books the size of the one you are reading. Trying to fish out a single specific gene from the entire genome would thus be akin to hunting down a few dozen lines from a several-thousand-volume set of encyclopedias! The task is made even more complicated by the fact that only about three percent of the DNA in the human genome is used to spell out genes; the purpose of the remaining DNA is largely unknown at present.

Breaking DNA into smaller pieces is not really the problem. Forcing solutions of DNA through very small holes at high pressure will readily shear it into smaller fragments. By controlling the shearing conditions, the average size of the fragments can be kept within a workable range. But there are a number of serious problems with this approach. The first

* Because of the double-stranded nature of DNA, lengths of DNA are marked off not in individual nucleotides, but in pairs, to account for both chains. For historical reasons, mol-ecular biologists refer to these as "base pairs" (abbreviated "bp"), rather than nucleotide pairs, in reference to the "base" component of each nucleotide (see Figure 1-6.) We will use the notation "bp" or "kbp" (kilobase pairs) from this point on when referring to lengths of DNA fragments.

problem comes with finding which of these fragments contains the gene of interest. Other biological molecules are often separated on the basis of their chemical properties, such as charge or hydrophobicity. But DNA is made up of only four different nucleotides; the chemical properties of any one gene are not going to be noticeably different from any other gene. The fragments resulting from mechanical disruption would be of different sizes, and it is certainly possible to separate DNA fragments on the basis of size. But the problem is that breaking up DNA by shearing is a random process. The same batch of DNA put through the same shearing process three times in a row would produce three different random batches of fragments. There would be no way of knowing which fragment a given gene would be associated with.

This problem was solved in a spectacularly successful way in the late 1960s and early 1970s when several investigators (most notably Hamilton Smith and Dan Nathans at Johns Hopkins University) began characterizing a unique type of DNA-cutting enzyme from bacteria called *restriction endonucleases*. These are enzymes used by bacteria to cut up any foreign DNA (bacteriophage DNA, for example) that might somehow cross their boundaries — there is no surer way to cripple a biological invader than to chew up its DNA! The very useful property of these enzymes is that they do not cut up DNA randomly, like the DNAse used as a medicine to help clear mucus from CF patients. Rather, they cleave DNA only at certain highly specific sites (called *restriction sites*) specified by particular sequences of nucleotides. About a hundred of these nucleases have been characterized to date, each from a different bacterial strain, and each with its own recognition sequence. The enzymes are usually named for the bacterial strain from which they are isolated. EcoRI, for example, was the first restriction enzyme ("RI") isolated from the common gut bacterium E. coli. EcoRI will always cut DNA whenever it encounters the nucleotide sequence GAATTC. Note that the sequence of nucleotides on the opposite strand at this site is the same, but running in the opposite direction: CTTAAG. Such *palindromic sequences* are a characteristic of many restriction enzymes. The enzyme cuts both strands, making a complete break in the DNA. Wherever this nucleotide sequence is found in the genome of an organism, EcoRI will cut its DNA. Because the nucleotide sequence for the DNA of a given organism is fixed, EcoRI will always cut the DNA of that organism in precisely the same way; it will always produce the same set of *restriction fragments* in the process.

The discovery of restriction nucleases was a major breakthrough in DNA technology, and perhaps more than any other single technical advance made the isolation and study of individual genes possible. The importance of this work was recognized with the award of the 1978 Nobel Prize in Physiology or Medicine to Dan Nathans, Hamilton Smith, and Werner Arber, a Swiss molecular biologist. The perceptive reader may well wonder how bacteria avoid cutting their own DNA with their potent restriction endonucleases. Each bacterium producing a restriction enzyme recognizing a particular nucleotide sequence also produces an enzyme that recognizes exactly the same sequence in its own DNA, but chemically alters it in such a way that the restriction enzyme cannot cleave it. The protective enzymes do not modify foreign DNA in the same way.

A defined sequence of four nucleotides will occur by chance once every two to three hundred nucleotides along an average stretch of DNA; a given sequence of six nucleotides will occur on average once every several thousand nucleotides. This is a very workable size range for most biochemical applications — DNA sequencing, for example. But how does one find the one or two fragments, among the millions that may be generated after digestion with a given nuclease, that contain the gene that one is looking for? This is a very critical procedure. The first step is to separate the fragments according to size by a process called *electrophoresis*. The way this is done is shown in Figure 5-2a. All of the DNA fragments generated by nuclease cleavage will have the same net electrical charge regardless of size. If they are loaded into a small rectangular well at one end of a thin coating of gel spread onto a glass plate, and subjected to an electrical field across the plate, the fragments will migrate through the gel according to size. The small fragments will move quickly and smoothly through the gel particles, while the larger fragments will be slowed down as they bump and squeeze through the gel. At the end of electrophoresis the fragments will be stretched out in a lane running down from the loading well, with the larger fragments at the top and the smaller fragments at the bottom. The fragments can be visualized in the gel using a DNA-staining dye called *ethidium bromide*. The great advantage of the nuclease digestion technique is that the same DNA sample digested with the same nuclease will always give exactly the same pattern of restriction fragments.

Somewhere among these fragments will be the one or two containing the gene of interest. How do we find them? The technique for doing this

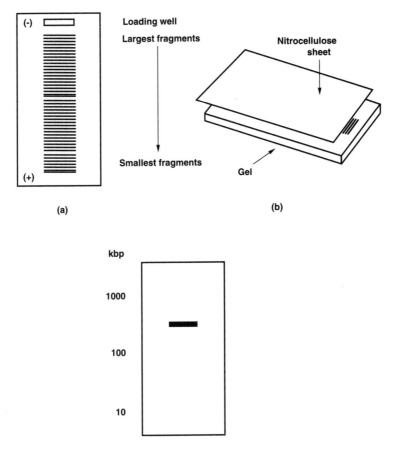

Figure 5-2. Southern blot.

is called a *Southern blot*, named after its originator, Edward Southern (Figure 5-2b). First, the DNA from an electrophoresis gel is transferred (blotted) onto a thin sheet of paper-like material called nitrocellulose; the pattern on the blot will be an exact mirror image of the fragment pattern on the gel. Next, the filter is incubated with a solution of highly radioactive, gene-specific probe. The generation of an appropriate DNA probe is one of the most critical steps in identifying and isolating genes. We will see how various probes are generated in subsequent chapters when we discuss specific disease-causing genes. Basically, a probe is a short DNA segment containing some portion of a gene. Since DNA is double-stranded, any DNA segment along the strand just opposite a given gene can serve as a probe for that gene. Because the probe (like the opposing DNA strand itself) is complementary to the gene, it will bind tightly to the gene through standard A-T, G-C pairing. Even a small piece of DNA used as a probe will bind tightly to either small or large pieces of a gene on a Southern blot. The probe is tagged either with a radioactive atom or a fluorescent molecule. After thoroughly washing away any unbound probe, the blot is laid on a sheet of X-ray film. Radioactive emissions from the bound probe will show up as black lines on the developed film, marking the position of the fragments bearing the gene in question. Fluorescent emissions are deteced electronically. The identity of a particular band is usually denoted by its size in kbp, as determined by comparison with size standards run with each gel.

Cloning DNA

The amount of any given DNA fragment that can be isolated from even large amounts of tissue is far too small for direct study. It is thus necessary to expand these DNA fragments a million- or even a billion-fold for laboratory work and eventual clinical use; that is the purpose of *DNA cloning*. The ability to clone DNA was one of the most valuable, if unanticipated, side benefits of the discovery of restriction endonucleases.

The idea behind DNA cloning is rather simple. As shown in Figure 5-3, when a sample of DNA is first digested with certain endonucleases, the two strands of the DNA are cut in a staggered fashion, creating what are called "sticky ends." All of the sticky ends generated by a given endonuclease are always the same: for example, the nuclease EcoRI always generates AATT at one end of each double-stranded piece, and TTAA at the other end. The reason these are called sticky ends is that under the right conditions the ends of any two pieces generated by the same nuclease can overlap with each other, creating a semi-stable complex. (Note that AATT and TTAA are complementary by the A-T, G-C rule.) This complex can be "locked in" with a special enzyme called DNA ligase. So a sample of DNA could be digested with EcoRI, stirred around a bit, and then stitched together with ligase into a completely random string of DNA fragments.

But one can do something infinitely more clever and useful than that: one can insert nuclease-generated fragments of human DNA into *cloning vectors*. An example of a cloning vector is the tiny, circular pieces of double-stranded DNA growing in bacteria called *plasmids*. Plasmids are not

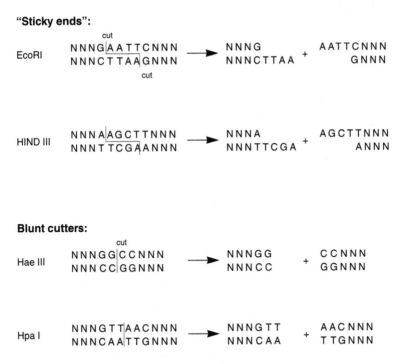

"Sticky ends":

                    cut
          NNNG|AATTCNNN   NNNG   AATTCNNN
EcoRI   ──────▶   +
          NNNCTTAA|GNNN   NNNCTTAA   GNNN
                    cut

          NNNA|AGCTTNNN   NNNA   AGCTTNNN
HIND III   ──────▶   +
          NNNTTCGA|ANNN   NNNTTCGA   ANNN

Blunt cutters:

                  cut
          NNNGG|CCNNN   NNNGG   CCNNN
Hae III   ──────▶   +
          NNNCC|GGNNN   NNNCC   GGNNN

          NNNGTT|AACNNN   NNNGTT   AACNNN
Hpa I   ──────▶   +
          NNNCAA|TTGNNN   NNNCAA   TTGNNN

Figure 5-3. Examples of restriction enzyme cuts.

part of the bacterial DNA proper; they are more like a permanent, in-dwelling virus that the bacteria replicate when they replicate their own DNA during cell division. (Geneticists refer to such extrachromosomal pieces of DNA as *episomal DNA*.) The plasmids usually contain some gene that the bacteria have found useful, but do not have in their own genomes. Therefore they replicate the plasmid as if it were their own DNA, and pass it on to the next generation. Scientists have learned to take marvelous advantage of this biological quirk.

In the laboratory, plasmids can be easily isolated separately from the bacterial "chromosome" because of the huge difference in size. If a sample of human DNA is digested with EcoRI, and a plasmid is cut open with the same enzyme, each sample will have the same sticky ends (Figure 5-4.) If the two samples are mixed together, they will form randomly assembled, semi-stable complexes. Many of the complexes will be human-human or plasmid-plasmid, but some proportion of them will be human-plasmid: a fragment of human DNA inserted into what can now be thought of as a plasmid vector. When these are all ligated and *transfected*

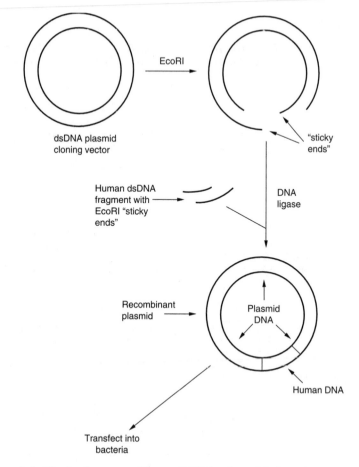

dsDNA plasmid
cloning vector

EcoRI

"sticky
ends"

Human dsDNA
fragment with
EcoRI "sticky
ends"

DNA
ligase

Recombinant
plasmid

Plasmid
DNA

Human DNA

Transfect into
bacteria

Figure 5-4. Cloning fragments of human DNA in a bacterial plasmid.

into bacteria, some of the human-plasmid *recombinant DNA* will in fact be accepted by the bacteria and propagated just like normal plasmids. Bacteria divide very rapidly — under optimal conditions as often as every thirty minutes. Within a short time, a miniscule amount of human DNA grown in a plasmid vector can be expanded into very sizeable quantities.

The bacteria transfected with recombinant plasmids are initially distributed onto the surface of bacterial growth plates where they form individual colonies (Figure 5-5). Some of the bacteria will have no plasmid; some will have plasmids that have simply resealed into their original form; and some will have plasmids containing the selected piece of DNA. Each colony on the plate is derived from a single bacterium, and thus each

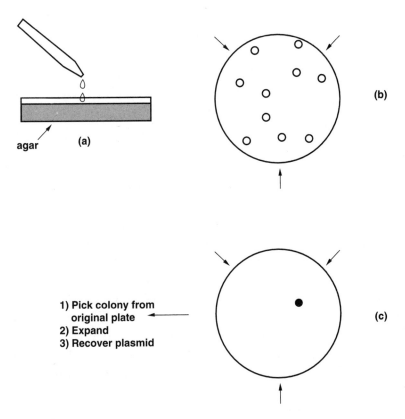

Figure 5-5. Screening bacterial colonies for human DNA. Bacteria transfected with plasmids containing a human DNA insert are dripped onto agar plates, spread out and allowed to grow overnight (a). To detect colonies containing the desired gene, a blot is made from the surface of the plate, with reference points carefully noted on the plate and blot (arrows.) The blot is then incubated with a radioactive or fluorescent probe specific for the human DNA fragment; only those colonies containing the fragment will "light up" by binding the probe, which can be detected on a piece of film pressed against the blot (c.) By using the reference arrows, the film can be placed over the original agar plate (b), and bacteria from the underlying colony can then be picked and grown in large quantities in flasks of bacterial growth medium.

member of a distinct colony is a true "clone" of a single starting bacterium, and will contain within it the identical recombinant plasmid. Each colony represents a different clone. When the colonies reach about one milimeter in size, they are "blotted" onto a nitrocellulose filter in a procedure similar to the Southern blotting procedure. The blot is then treated with chemicals to break open the bacteria and allow their DNA to interact with a probe made from the piece of human DNA that was originally cloned into the plasmid. Once a specific human DNA-containing plasmid has been thus identified, it can be picked off the plate and expanded into virtually unlimited quantities by standard bacterial growth techniques. It is a fairly simple operation at the end of the growth period to recover the plasmid from the bacteria, and to splice out the passenger gene.

In principle, any form of DNA can be inserted into bacterial vectors for expansion. DNA isolated directly from the genome (i.e., the DNA making up the chromosomes) is sometimes cloned for study. In other instances, it makes more sense to clone something called *complementary DNA (cDNA)*. In the 1970s, David Baltimore and Howard Temin, in a Nobel Prize-winning work, showed that certain viruses (called *retroviruses*) have an enzyme that can "reverse transcribe" RNA into DNA. Using this enzyme (called *reverse transcriptase*), it is possible to convert mRNA into its exact DNA "mirror image," cDNA. The initial cDNA, like mRNA, is single-stranded, but can readily be converted to a double-stranded form (ds-cDNA), which can then be inserted into bacterial vectors such as plasmids. If the cDNA to be cloned does not have sticky ends, it is possible simply to buy them and "paste" them on to the existing cDNA ends. It is also possible to introduce cDNA into cut vectors by so-called "blunt-end ligation."

One very useful application of cDNA cloning is the construction of a *cDNA library*. These libraries contain samples of all of the genes expressed in a particular cell type. All such genes will be represented by mRNA molecules being actively translated into protein within the cell. All of the mRNA from a particular cell line is converted to cDNA, and inserted into plasmids which are then transfected into bacteria. As with standard cloning techniques, the transfected bacteria are cloned onto bacterial growth plates. Individual colonies are picked, expanded slightly, and stored away as individual "volumes" in a library for future scanning with various probes. If the cell of origin was a liver cell, for example, one now has a cDNA library representing all the genes being actively expressed (i.e., transcribed into mRNA) in liver cells. These libraries are extremely useful in molecular biology. Finally, as we will see, the ds-cDNA form of a gene is usually the form of choice for gene therapy. With certain modifications to the cDNA, cells will be able to reconvert cDNA back into

Table 5-1. *DNA cloning vectors*

Cloning Vector	Upper Limit for DNA Inserts
Plasmids	10–12 kbp
Cosmids	35–45 kbp
Bacterial artificial chromosome (BAC)	250–300 kbp
Yeast artificial chromosome (YAC)	1,500–2,000 kbp

single-stranded mRNA, which can then be translated by the cell into the needed protein.

There is an upper limit to the amount of DNA that can be inserted into plasmids and, very often, as we will see later, researchers need to clone larger pieces. *Cosmids* are vectors made from a combination of viral and bacterial genomes that can accomodate about twice as much DNA as standard plasmids (Table 5-1.) Even larger amounts of DNA can be cloned by actually incorporating them into bacterial or yeast chromosomes, where they are replicated by the host cell during normal chromosomal replication.

One of the first things scientists usually want to do with a new sample of cloned DNA is to sequence it. As we said earlier, sequencing the gene is now the easiest way to gain information about the amino acid sequence of the corresponding protein. Either the genomic form of a gene or the cDNA form can be sequenced. Sequencing of the genomic form of a gene provides useful information about a gene's identity, as well as the regulation of its expression in the different cells. Details of how DNA sequencing is done are beyond the scope of this book, but the methods are now essentially automated, and large pieces of DNA can be sequenced in a very short time. The Human Genome Project, which we will discuss in a later chapter, has nothing less for its goal than obtaining the complete nucleotide sequence of the entire human genome. This project is expected to be completed by the year 2003.

One of the most important things to be learned about gene structure from DNA sequencing studies concerns certain regulatory elements found in front of (or "upstream of") each true gene (Figure 5-6). Just upstream of the "start codons" that mark the first letter of each gene, there are several *promoter sequences* that guide the enzymatic machinery involved in actually transcribing the gene. These elements, which are similar in nucleotide sequence for all genes, help the transcribing enzymes

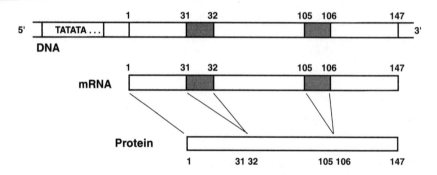

Figure 5-6. **The structure and proceessing of mammalian genes.** The first codon specifying an amino acid (1) is preceded by several stretches of DNA, such as the "TATA box" (a region rich in the A and T nucleotides), which help position the transcriptional machinery. "Exons" (shaded areas) are interrupted by "introns" (open areas) which have no coding function.

bind to the DNA and produce the all-important RNA transcripts that ultimately become mRNA. When scientists sequence their way through an unknown DNA region, the presence of promoter sequences is a good indication that the nucleotides that follow downstream contain an embedded gene. And when genes are transferred into cells in gene therapy, a promoter for the "passenger gene" must always be included.

A major surprise to come from the sequencing of genes was the presence, in animal cell DNA, of something called *introns*. In bacterial DNA, the nucleotide sequence of a given gene is exactly colinear with the protein it encodes. But genes from animal cells are different. The coding portion of a gene is broken up into several *exons*, which are physically separated by noncoding introns (see Figure 5-6). The sequences of introns have no relation to the coding sequences among which they are interspersed. While exon sequences for a given gene are highly conserved among closely related species, intron sequences for the same gene can vary greatly between even the most closely related species, and even within a species. The function of introns has been a matter of intense speculation ever since they were discovered, but their significance is still unclear. They are one of the contributing factors to a strange property of animal cell DNA: only about three to five percent of the DNA codes for proteins. The rest of the DNA, like introns, is of largely unknown function. It is often referred to as "nonsense" DNA, although that is unlikely to be an accurate description of its true biological role. Transcription of the gene

Table 5-2. *Some examples of recombinant human proteins approved for clinical use.*

Protein	Use
Insulin	Treating Type-1 diabetes
Human growth hormone	Treating dwarfism
Tissue plasminogen activator (TPA)	Dissolving clots in heart attack and stroke
Erythropoeitin	Stimulate red blood cell production
Interferon gamma	Boost immune resistance
Granulocyte colony stimulating factor	Increase production of white blood cells
Interleukin-2	Stimulate the immune system
Monoclonal antibodies	Cancer diagnosis

results in production of an mRNA that lacks most of the upstream sequences, but retains the introns. (The numbers above the DNA and mRNA in Figure 5-6 refer to the amino acid position in the final protein product.) Before leaving the nucleus, the mRNA is further processed to remove the introns and any other remaining non-coding sequences; the final protein product consists only of the amino acids specified in the exonic DNA codons.

The ability to isolate and clone individual human genes or cDNA provided one of the first benefits of molecular medicine: the ability to produce large quantities of highly pure human proteins for therapeutic use. Proteins produced from foreign genes cloned into a producer cell line are called *recombinant proteins*. One of the first and most important of such proteins was human insulin for use in treating diabetes. This important hormone was first produced in bacteria in 1978, and was approved for use in humans in 1982. Today there are literally hundreds of such proteins available for clinical use (Table 5-2.) In many instances recombinant human proteins have all but displaced the animal proteins formerly used, such as bovine or porcine insulin. Although initially very expensive to produce, evolving technology and economies of scale have made many recombinant proteins economically competitive as well as therapeutically superior.

While expression of cloned human genes in bacteria is possible and has some advantages in terms of large-scale production and lower costs, most recombinant proteins intended for use in humans—especially those intended for gene therapy—are produced in mammalian cell lines. Bacterial cells tend to degrade recombinant proteins, but more importantly often do not fold them properly after synthesis. Untangling them and getting them to refold properly is very time-consuming and expensive. Also, bacteria do not know how to add carbohydrate groups to proteins, which are vital for the function of many human proteins. Continuously-growing animal or human cell lines, with strange names such as Chinese hamster ovary cells or baby hamster kidney cells, can carry out all of these functions properly, given an appropriately engineered human gene. Such cells grow much more slowly than bacteria, and require more expensive culture medium for growth, but the absolute integrity of the final product justifies the additional cost. The cDNA form of human genes, with promoters and other information related to the final processing of the resulting mRNA spliced onto them, are grown in bacterial plasmids and then introduced into a mammalian cell line for expression of the protein product. The protein is harvested (often from the liquid culture medium in which the cells are grown) and purified extensively for use. Because the proteins are produced in mammalian cells, the possibility of contaminating, potentially harmful bacterial products is bypassed completely. Virtually any human protein for which the gene has been isolated, and for which there is a sufficiently large market to justify the production costs, can be produced by this method.

Gene Therapy: Transferring Genes into Human Cells

Once a gene responsible for a particular disease has been isolated and cloned, numerous preliminary studies must be carried out before it is ready for use in gene therapy. The most important of these studies is that of devising a strategy for getting the gene into cells and, once inside, getting it transcribed and translated. With a few important exceptions, simply mixing genes with cells will not work. Although animal cells will take up nucleic acids to some extent, the efficiency is in most cases much too low for this approach to be of any practical use. Molecular biologists thus use various *transducing vectors* for genes, of which two general types have proved successful: viruses and liposomes.

Viral Delivery Vectors. Viruses have many highly desirable characteristics for use in delivering genes to cells, not the least of which is that they have been selected over millions of years of coevolution with animal cells to do just that: transfer their own nucleic acid genome (either DNA or RNA) into cells for processing into protein products. Viruses are extremely adept at binding to cell membranes and passing their genomes through them — no mean feat from a chemical point of view. It is relatively straightforward to insert an additional gene, even a human gene, into the viral genome. Once inside the cell, viruses have various strategies for getting their genomes to be "read" by the *transduced* host cell (Figure 5-7). Any foreign gene included in the viral genome will also be read by the host cell, as long as the gene is preceded by an appropriate promoter.

Among the more useful viral vectors for carrying a passenger gene into an animal cell are the *retroviruses*. Retroviruses are single-stranded RNA viruses that, immediately after entering a cell, convert their RNA into double-stranded DNA. This ds-DNA state of the viral genome is referred to as the *provirus*, because it inserts into the host cell DNA where it directs the production of single-stranded RNA molecules that are ultimately packaged into new retroviruses. Because the viral DNA is stably inserted into the host genome, viral production can go on indefinitely — unless, of course, the virus kills the cell, which is what happens with HIV, the retrovirus causing AIDS. The ability of retroviruses to insert their DNA into the host cell genome is what makes them so attractive for transducing vectors. The provirus form of the virus can be isolated, cut open with a restriction nuclease, and a ds-cDNA copy of a human gene can be inserted.

Because many of the retroviruses attractive for use as gene delivery vectors are associated with disease, the virus must first be disabled before transfer into human beings. This is done by removing key genes needed for viral replication. Retroviruses have relatively few genes, and most of these can be removed from the provirus before inserting the passenger gene to be delivered. But this creates a problem: If the virus is rendered unable to replicate, how is it possible to grow up enough copies of the virus and its passenger gene to use for gene therapy? This can be done by using a "packaging cell" (Figure 5-8). These are cells that have been given copies of the missing viral genes so that they can supply the proteins necessary for packaging the altered viral genome. Viruses produced by pack-

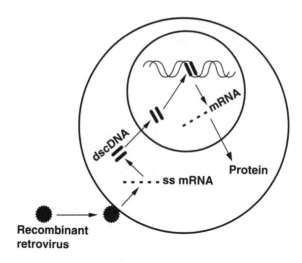

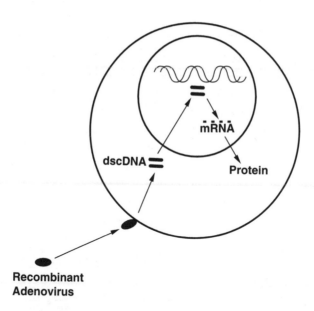

Figure 5-7. **Viral vectors for transduction of foreign DNA into cells.** After conversion of a retroviral genome to dscDNA form (also called the "provirus"), the retroviral genes together with any passenger genes are inserted into the host cell's DNA, where they can remain more or less indefinitely. For most other viruses, like adenovirus (bottom), the viral and passenger genes remain free in the nucleus as an "episome", and are eventually lost.

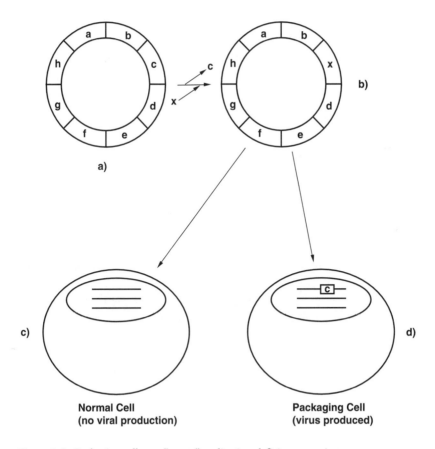

Figure 5-8. Packaging cells can "rescue" replication-deficient retroviruses.
The retroviral genome shown in (a) is selected for use as gene delivery vector. A gene needed by the virus for replication in a host cell ("c") is removed, and replaced with the gene to be delivered ("x"). At this stage, only small amounts of altered virus are made, essentially in test tubes; the problem is now to produce the quantities of altered virus needed for large-scale transduction experiments. The recombinant virus (b) is able to infect both normal and packaging cells, but because of the missing viral gene it cannot replicate in the normal cell. However, in a separate experiment a copy of the missing viral gene has been integrated into the DNA of a normal cell to make it into a packaging cell; in this cell, the protein needed by the virus to reproduce ("c") is now present, and viral reproduction on a large scale can take place. But the viruses thus produced still lack the crucial replication gene. When they infect normal cells, the recombinant genome is incorporated into the host genome. The passenger gene can be "read" by the host cell to make the corresponding protein, but the virus per se cannot replicate.

aging cells are able to infect human cells, convert the recombinant viral RNA genome to a proviral ds-DNA form, and insert the proviral DNA into the host cell genome. The passenger gene inserted into the virus will be read, and the corresponding protein produced, as if it were a normal part of the host cell; however, there is not sufficient viral information to direct the production of infectious viral particles.

Retroviruses do have disadvantages as transduction vectors. First of all, as with any viral vector, there is always the fear that all of the genes necessary for viral replication may not have been removed from all of the viral genomes used. With experience and the highly refined technology available today, this has become of decreasing concern. A second concern is that retroviruses generally infect only rapidly dividing cells. This is not a problem if the target is bone marrow or most blood cells, which either are dividing or can readily be made to do so, but it renders retroviruses unsuitable for carrying genes into most other cell types. A third and more serious problem is the possibility of causing the targeted cell to become cancerous. Retroviral proviruses insert themselves randomly into the host genome, and on occasion right into the middle of a functional gene. Since functional genes comprise only about three percent of our DNA, this does not happen often. If the disrupted gene is critical to cell function, the altered cell will probably die and disappear from view. But if a retrovirus disrupts one of the genes whose function is to prevent a cell from entering into unscheduled cell division, the loss of this control could lead to cancer. Moreover, if inserted into the host DNA near a gene that causes cancer when turned on, the promoter used to drive transcription of the passenger gene could activate the cancer gene and trigger development of a tumor. For many retroviruses such *insertional mutagenesis* happens only rarely, but for others it is a constant concern and a reason not to use retroviral vectors except for diseases that are life threatening.

To deliver genes to nondividing cells, the most commonly used viral vectors are derived from adenoviruses. Adenoviruses are double-stranded DNA viruses that ordinarily cause mild flulike symptoms in humans. Adenovirus DNA can be cut open with restriction enzymes, key genes required for viral reproduction removed, and a ds-cDNA copy of a gene inserted. The recombinant virus will readily infect a human cell. However, unlike retroviruses, adenoviruses do not insert their DNA into the host genome. The recombinant viral DNA enters the cell nucleus where it remains a separate episomal DNA element (see Figure 5-7). This is one of the major advantages—and at the same time one of the major drawbacks—of adenovirus as a delivery vector. Because the new genome remains episomal, there is no danger of a mutational event caused by vector insertion into the host DNA. However, the episomal DNA will be degraded by the cell over time, and will have to be readministered. This is not necessarily a limiting problem, as we will see in the cystic fibrosis gene therapy trials.

A second and potentially more serious problem with adenoviruses as delivery vectors, and one that is exacerbated by the need for repeated administrations, is that adenovirus provokes a rather strong host immune response that can lead to destruction of transfected cells. Adenovirus is much larger than the retroviruses, and its genome encodes a large number of virus-specific proteins. While it is possible to remove enough genes to cripple viral reproduction in an infected host cell, it is not possible to remove all or even most adenoviral genes, and the proteins encoded by the remaining genes stimulate the immune system to attack transfected cells. The more often it is administered, the stronger the immune response. Scientists are currently working on ways to make the adenovirus less *immunogenic*.

Liposomal Delivery Vectors. Liposomes are simply cell-membranelike envelopes into which nucleic acids or other materials can be packaged. Although made of natural materials, liposomes per se are not biological in origin; they are made in the laboratory from fat (lipid) molecules arranged in such a way that they make tiny spheres. Materials present in the reaction mixture where liposomes are formed become trapped in these spheres. This fact has been taken advantage of in recent years to deliver many different drugs; DNA should be no different. In this case the gene of interest (with appropriate promoter sequences) is usually carried in a plasmid within the liposome. Such plasmids can be engineered to hold larger pieces of foreign DNA than normal, another advantage of liposomes.

The chemical composition of liposomes is selected to resemble the membranes of cells. When mixed with living cells under appropriate conditions, the liposomes can fuse with the cells' plasma membranes, emptying their contents into the cell interiors. In some cases cells will take up small liposomes almost as if they were trying to eat them; once inside, the DNA can fuse with internal membranes and escape into the cytoplasm.

In either case, DNA delivered in this fashion can enter the nucleus, but it remains episomal and thus must be periodically readministered.

While definitely less efficient than viruses, liposomes have the great advantage that they are not themselves toxic or pathogenic, and they do not provoke a host immune response. Moreover, like adenoviruses, liposomes do not require dividing cells with which to fuse. A disadvantage of liposomes is that they must generally be applied directly to the cells with which they are intended to fuse. As we will see, this is fine for diseases such as CF, where the gene-containing liposomes can be dripped or sprayed into the airways. In general, however, liposomes cannot be injected into the blood stream to reach other tissues and organs, because they have no way of getting out of the bloodstream to reach their targets. Interestingly, the blood vessels serving many tumors are "leaky," and liposomes may preferentially leave the bloodstream at the site of a tumor. This offers some interesting possibilities for treatment of cancer, including gene therapy treatments, as we shall see.

Because of their advantages in terms of safety, a great deal of research is currently underway to improve the efficiency with which liposomes can deliver DNA to cells. Alterations in the lipid composition can affect the length of time they remain in the body, and their efficiency in both drug trapping and fusion with target cells. Scientists are now trying to build targeting molecules into the surface of liposomes to guide them to specific tissues and organs. This could have a favorable effect on efficiency of liposome delivery of both drugs and DNA.

Building more efficient delivery vectors to suit specific needs is one of the most important areas of research in gene therapy, and will be an important factor in the long-term success of molecular medicine. But now it is time to take a look at the present state of the art in gene therapy, using the tools and techniques already at hand.

6

The Journey Begins

The Clinical Trials for ADA-SCID

Gene Therapy: The First Halting Steps

The possibilities for applying the emerging techniques of molecular biology to human gene therapy were appreciated by a handful of people as early as the late 1960s, although at that time no one had the slightest idea of how human genes might be isolated. The first human gene would not even be cloned for another dozen or so years. But there were tantalizing clues of what might lie ahead. In the 1960s, a physician-scientist named Stanfield Rogers at the Oak Ridge National Laboratories made an extraordinary observation with the common wart-causing *Shope papilloma virus*. One of the genes carried by this virus encodes an enzyme called *arginase*, which degrades excess amounts of the amino acid arginine. In addition to its role as a building block of protein, arginine also plays a role of its own as an intermediate in the processing of nitrogenous wastes in the body. Rogers noted that in rabbits infected with the *Shope* virus, the levels of arginine in the blood were unusually low. This did not particularly bother the rabbits; in fact high levels of arginine can be toxic. But what struck Rogers was that a viral gene appeared to be carrying out an important metabolic function in a rabbit. Rogers became curious as to whether any of the laboratory personnel handling the infected rabbits had themselves become infected with the virus, not an uncommon occurrence in the laboratory. Upon removing blood samples from people in the laboratory, he found out that not only had some of them become infected (not a serious event in itself; the immune system can easily control papilloma infections), but they also had extremely low levels of arginine in their bloodstreams.

This was a profound and profoundly interesting finding. It showed that genes carried as part of a viral genome could alter normal physiological processes in a human being. Rogers immediately recognized the potential of viruses for delivering genes to human beings. A few years later, he came upon an opportunity to test his thinking in a direct way on two young patients suffering from the toxic effects of excess arginine in their systems. He deliberately exposed them to the Shope virus in an attempt to reduce their arginine levels. Hoping to err on the side of caution, he used amounts too low to be effective, and neither good nor harm came of his experiment. But Rogers himself was severely criticized for taking what some saw as an unwarranted risk based on premature and less-than-compelling data. Nevertheless, the overall lesson about the ability of viruses to carry genes into human beings would not be forgotten.

The reality of gene therapy was brought a step closer a decade later, with an experiment that would again be roundly criticized by the scientific community. The first human gene to be isolated and cloned (in 1977) was that for β-globin, one of the subunits of hemoglobin, the oxygen-carrying molecule of red blood cells. Defects in the β-globin gene can cause serious diseases such as sickle-cell anemia and thalassemia. Just two years after the β-globin gene had been isolated, a physician at UCLA, working with a basic scientist at his institution, tried introducing the gene into mouse bone-marrow cells using a viral vector. The experiment worked; moreover, when the altered bone-marrow cells were put back into mice, there was evidence that they survived and that the added gene was functioning in vivo. The researchers then applied to their university's Human Subjects Protection Committee for permission to try the same thing in human patients with thalassemia. Unable to get permission from his home institution, the team's physician member proceeded to recruit patients suffering from thalassemia in institutions outside the U.S. Several patients had samples of their bone marrow removed, exposed to the vector containing the β-globin gene, and reinfused into their bloodstream. The experiment failed to alter the course of their disease, although the patients appeared to suffer no harm from the procedure. The physician was taken severely to task by his institution, by the federal government, and by the international scientific community.

The results of this first attempt at gene therapy using cloned DNA, and the overwhelmingly negative response it engendered, gave caution to those eager to seize the day and be the first to make the dream of molecular medicine come true. But it also became abundantly clear to everyone who was watching that the technology for gene therapy was now in hand, and that it would only be a matter of time before genuine clinical trials for gene therapy would begin.

Paving the Way: Human Clinical Trials

Clinical trials represent the transition phase between highly promising basic laboratory research on a new drug or treatment method, and the general release of that drug or treatment to the larger medical community for use in standard therapy. Just a few decades ago, clinical trials were generally informally organized studies carried out by physicians, usually in collaboration with drug companies, to test a new drug, medical device, or clinical procedure. These studies were often not standardized, lacked important controls, and did not pay attention to proper statistical analysis of data. As a result, many clinical trials produced data of little real value. Yet patients were put at risk during such trials, and patients subsequently treated by drugs or devices approved for general use by these clinical trials were also, unknowingly, at risk.

In the 1970s, the federal government began formulating specific sets of guidelines for clinical trials, and today all new drugs and invasive medical devices are subjected to rigorously controlled clinical tests before they are made available for general clinical use. Clinical trials in the U. S. are now overseen by the Food and Drug Administration (FDA). The FDA has final authority for approving new drugs and invasive medical devices for manufacture, marketing, and general use by the medical community. Clinical trials are most often carried out in university medical centers under the guidance of physicians who also have strong basic science backgrounds, or have basic science consultants as part of the overall clinical trial team. In most cases, a potential manufacturer or marketer of a new drug or procedure will be an active partner in clinical trials, providing the drug itself and any other needed materials and generally underwriting their costs.

All institutions sponsoring clinical trials must have an internal Institutional Review Board (IRB) to review clinical trial proposals before they are even submitted for FDA approval. It is the job of the IRB (called the Human Subjects Protection Committee in some institutions) to carry out an initial assessment of the scientific soundness of the proposal, and to be sure that the data collection and analysis procedures are valid and meaningful. It is also the IRB's responsibility to determine that the proposed patient population is appropriate for the aims of the trial, and that proper patient informed consent procedures will be followed.

At first, the human genes proposed for use in gene therapy might not seem to fit the category of "new drug." However, these genes will be delivered in viral or chemical vectors, they will eventually be prepared for use by standard manufacturing procedures, and we know little about the long-term effects of introducing extraneous DNA into human beings. These factors suggest that the same caution should be exercised with DNA as with any other new drug until such time as the safety and efficacy of each procedure has been established beyond reasonable doubt.

Before a clinical trial can begin, the FDA must see compelling evidence from laboratory studies that a proposed new drug or procedure can actually do what its creators hope to achieve in humans. This *preclinical phase* of testing generally involves laboratory experiments with human cells grown outside the body, used to gain insight into potential toxicity and to be sure that the drug will actually work in humans. The next step is to test the drug or procedure in animals. This work often begins with rats and mice, for reasons of economy, the large backlog of experience with these animals, and knowledge of how their physiology compares with humans. A very useful animal model that finds increasing use in drug testing is the so-called *nude mouse*. Nude mice have a genetic defect that prevents them from immunologically rejecting human cells and tissues. (A closely linked defect prevents them from developing fur; hence the "nude" designation.) It is thus possible to transplant into nude mice a small piece of the human tissue a new drug is supposed to affect, to inject that drug into the mice, and to monitor the drug's effect on the human tissue under "in vivo" conditions. In some cases it may be appropriate to test the drug further on a larger animal before testing in humans, but increasingly the nude-mouse model has been able to satisfy federal regulators.

Ultimately, of course, any new drug or procedure must be tested on human beings to be absolutely certain that it is safe, and that it has the effect intended by its developers. The FDA has developed very strict guidelines for conducting human clinical trials. The first principle of any clinical trial is fully informed consent of the human subjects who will participate in the trial. Patients (or their families, in those cases where patients are gravely ill) must clearly understand the experimental nature of the procedures they will undergo, the possible dangers they may face, and how the information gathered will be used. They must not be mis-led about potential benefits or improvements to their underlying dis-ease. Confidentiality of the information gathered during the trial must be assured. A copy of information provided to each patient is reviewed by the FDA as part of the overall approval process for any new clinical trial.

Clinical trials are typically divided into four phases. Each phase is reviewed while it proceeds, and each phase must be completed and approved before the next phase can begin. Although the exact description of each phase may be slightly different for each new drug or procedure, the following general guidelines apply to the majority of trials conducted.

Phase I. The principal purpose of a Phase I clinical trial is to gather infor-mation on safety of the proposed drug or procedure in human beings. In the case of a new drug (including DNA used for gene therapy) investiga-tors will look at things such as how long the drug remains in the system, whether its properties change once it is inside a human body, and whether it causes any measurable side effects, either as reported by the subject or as detected in laboratory tests. Usually a range of doses of the drug will be tested, guided by previous toxicity tests in animals. However, in most Phase I trials patients will only receive a single administration of an exper-imental drug. The clinical tests may be carried out on persons with the disease for which the drug is intended, or occasionally they may be car-ried out on healthy volunteers. If the drug is to be tested on persons with active disease, it is usually patients with very advanced disease, who have failed to respond to standard current therapies, who are enrolled in the trials first. The number of patients involved in Phase I studies is small, no more than the number required to get statistically believable data for the points under study (typically a few to a few dozen individuals).

Phase II. While the effectiveness of a new drug on the condition it is intended to treat (its *efficacy*) is usually monitored during a Phase I trial, efficacy is really the focus of Phase II trials. Dosage and toxicity limits derived from Phase I studies are used to design a larger-scale trial to begin assessing the value of the new drug or treatment as compared to existing treatments. Patients with less advanced stages of disease may be entered into Phase II trials, and may receive multiple administrations of the drug. Patients are still closely monitored for toxicity or side effects of any kind. (Healthy volunteers do not participate in clinical trials beyond Phase I.) Somewhat larger numbers of patients may be involved, in the range of a few dozen to a hundred or so. Numerous controls are usually built into Phase II trials, including placebo treatments for some patient groups, patients with no previous treatment for their disease, patients receiving various combinations of standard therapies, and so forth.

Phase III. If drug efficacy with acceptable side effects can be established in Phase I and II trials, larger numbers of patients (hundreds to thousands) are enrolled in Phase III trials, usually in a variety of clinical settings (community hospitals as well as university medical centers). Additional data on the interaction of the new drug with existing drugs used to treat the disease are gathered. Information gathered in Phase III will eventually be used to instruct physicians about use of the new drug; toxicity is still closely monitored. The drug developer will usually apply for formal approval from the FDA to market the new drug after successful conclusion of Phase III trials.

Phase IV. Occasionally, the FDA will approve a new drug for general use, but require the manufacturer to continue monitoring the effects of the drug for a limited period after general release. In Phase IV trials, the drug may be extended to slightly different patient populations than those studied in earlier trials, dosages may be altered, or the drug tested in combinations with other previously approved drugs. The drug may also be extended for use in related conditions not specified in the original trials.

Although viewed by some as unnecessarily rigid and time consuming, there is no question that clinical trials carried out in the U.S. today produce sound, scientifically meaningful information about proposed new drugs, devices, and procedures, and protect the patients involved in the trials. By the time human gene therapy was ready for clinical trials, the steps necessary for approval were fairly well defined. But, as we will see, gene therapy introduced some new complications and concerns that at least initially made the approval process even more difficult than it had been in the past.

Isolation of the Gene for ADA

The involvement of ADA deficiency in one form of SCID had been appreciated from the early 1970s, and the disease was recognized as a single-gene defect almost as soon as it was described. Moreover, long before the gene was cloned and sequenced, it was also realized that the variable ADA-SCID severities observed clinically would likely be due to different mutations in a single, common gene.

The gene encoding ADA was one of the earlier human genes to be isolated and cloned for study. Three separate laboratories published the gene sequence in 1983. By that time several strategies had been developed for going after a gene that had never been isolated before. It is never easy; the degree of difficulty depends upon how much information is available about the gene or its product before starting. For example, in the 1950s scientists began isolating and sequencing proteins. As we saw in Chapter 3, getting the complete amino acid sequence of a protein is a daunting task, and can take years. Nevertheless, by the time restriction nucleases became available in the 1970s, which made isolating individual genes possible, the complete amino acid sequences of quite a few proteins were known, and partial sequences were available for a good many more. Knowing an amino acid sequence, and using the genetic code, it is possible to work backwards and predict the nucleic acid sequence of the corresponding gene. That information can then be used to chemically synthesize a complementary DNA probe that will detect the gene on a Southern blot.

That was one of the approaches used to identify the gene for ADA. One laboratory had isolated the human ADA protein in the late 1970s, and by the early 1980s had obtained enough amino acid sequence data on the purified protein to predict a region that seemed likely to be useful as a probe. A stretch of DNA consisting of seventeen nucleic acids (a "17-mer") was selected based on minimal predicted codon ambiguity (the confusion that can arise from the fact that more than one codon can specify a given amino acid). Even with a relative minimum of ambiguous codons, however, a total of sixty-four different 17-mer probes had to be synthesized to cover all possible combinations. These probes were used to screen a cDNA library made from human T cells, where the ADA gene was known to be expressed in high concentrations. The clones reactive with the probe mixture were then expanded, and the cDNA inserts isolated and sequenced. (Once a cDNA has actually been isolated, the cDNA itself often becomes the probe of choice for future work.)

At the time all of this was done, the possibility of using cloned DNA for gene therapy still seemed to most researchers a distant goal; the main purpose of cloning the ADA gene was to get more information on the relationship of genetic mutations to protein function. The usefulness of cloned portions of the gene as probes for genetic screening of at-risk populations was, however, immediately recognized. But within a short time, the possibility of using the newly isolated ADA gene for the first human gene therapy trials was under serious consideration. One of the first to make such a formal proposal was W. French Anderson, a physician-scientist at the National Institutes of Health. Anderson had been among the pioneers in pushing other physicians and research scientists to pursue the possibilities of applying recombinant DNA technology to the treatment of human genetic disorders. He had trained with Marshall Nirenberg, and had been part of the team that isolated the second human gene, α-globin, in 1977. Anderson recognized that since ADA-SCID could be cured by a bone-marrow transplant, the only critical locus for the ADA gene in this disease must be in a bone-marrow cell, or in a cell derived from bone marrow. Moreover, since heterozygotes are perfectly normal, a single copy of a "good" ADA gene within the critical cell type must be sufficient to correct the underlying defect. ADA-SCID seemed made for gene therapy.

By 1987 Anderson had prepared an initial proposal for clinical trials using the cloned human ADA gene to treat ADA-SCID patients. But first, Anderson had to clear his proposal through one of the most feared governmental regulatory agencies: the Recombinant DNA Advisory Committee. This committee, which oversees all federally funded research involving recombinant DNA, is referred to by all who go before it simply by its acronym: "the RAC."

The involvement of the RAC in clinical trials using recombinant DNA grew out of a defining moment in the history of molecular biology. Scientists began using restriction nucleases almost as soon as they became available in the early 1970s to make recombinant DNA molecules. Initial experiments involved nothing more than working out the conditions for cutting and stitching together pieces of DNA from various sources in test tubes. But before long scientists were eager to move on to more interesting possibilities. Some began carrying out experiments involving intact genomes removed from microorganisms such as bacteria and viruses. The first biologically functional recombinant DNA molecule was made by Herb Boyer and Stanley Cohen in 1973. They had placed a toad gene in a bacterial plasmid, and introduced the plasmid into a bacterial host strain; the bacteria promptly began making the corresponding toad protein. Paul Berg, a colleague of Boyer and Cohen and a pioneer in molecular biology, also carried out experiments recombining DNA from the genomes of different bacterial viruses (phage) that infect the common bacterium *E. coli*. Additionally, he had begun recombining phage genomes with portions of the genome of a virus called SV-40, which causes cancer in monkeys.

The resulting recombinant genomes were, in effect, totally new life forms, never before seen among organisms that had evolved naturally over eons of time. The problem is that *E. coli* lives, among other places, in the human gut. How would these new life forms, the recombinant phage, behave inside people? The new experiments with recombinant DNA were closely followed and widely known, and they were beginning to make some scientists slightly nervous. No one had ever before tampered with the genome of a living organism. When the resulting genome was associated with an organism that can infect human beings — and especially when it carried genes from a cancer-causing virus — it was felt that such tamperings needed a fuller discussion by the wider scientific community. There was no evidence that such experiments were in fact dangerous, but the suggestion was made that Berg and others should suspend further experimentation until everyone could get together for a talk.

The meeting to discuss the implications and possible risks of recombining the DNA of living organisms took place at the Asilomar Conference Center near Monterey, California, in 1974. All of the major laboratories working with recombinant DNA were invited, along with representatives of the federal agencies funding such research. To forestall any possible charges of a scientific elite meeting behind closed doors to decide the biological fate of humanity, the press was invited to participate. Many issues, some highly emotional as well as scientific, were aired in the formal sessions. But to an even larger extent discussions took place over meals, in the lodge where people gathered in the evenings, and in strolls along the spectacular adjoining beaches. Would the creation of recombinant genomes interfere with normal evolutionary processes? Do human beings have the right to reach into nature and create new life? Is that interfering with divine purpose? Could these organisms eventually have any military (i.e., biological warfare) applications?

Out of this meeting came a proposal to ask the prestigious National Academy of Sciences to establish a committee to review the current status of recombinant DNA technology, and to advise the government whether and how such research using this technology might need to be regulated. Paul Berg himself, as a member of the Academy, chaired the resulting committee. Berg's committee ultimately recommended that the National Institutes of Health establish a permanent Recombinant DNA Advisory Committee, which was formed almost immediately. Over the next two years, the RAC began formulating guidelines for carrying out recombinant DNA research funded by federal research grants. These guidelines were published by the NIH in 1976, and were adopted immediately by virtually all laboratories in the United States carrying out such research, however funded; the guidelines were also eventually adopted in one form or another by most governments throughout the world. The press was invited to observe every stage of this process, and played an important role in informing the public of what was taking place.

The early workings of the RAC dealt almost exclusively with safety issues for laboratory research. The major concern initially was that altered life forms would escape from laboratories and infect plants, animals or people on the outside. Guidelines for "containment" procedures, handling and storage of recombinant DNA, and other practical issues were disseminated to research laboratories throughout the country. Institutions sponsoring such research were required to establish Institutional Review Boards (IRBs) to ensure implementation of the RAC guidelines, and to assure that all applications for government research funding submitted to the NIH met RAC standards. Mindful of the furor that had attended the earlier forays in the direction of human gene therapy, the RAC also established a permanent Human Gene Therapy Subcommittee to carry out initial reviews of all research involving human genes, whether intended for therapeutic purposes or not.

The government later decided that any proposals to introduce DNA into human beings would also have to be subjected to clinical trials as defined by the Food and Drug Administration. Currently both the RAC and the FDA must approve clinical trials for gene therapy. There was a move on the part of some biotechnology companies and a few academics to have the RAC abolished, and to transfer sole authority for approving clinical trials to the FDA. However, after a thorough review of the workings of the RAC it was decided that its unique role in assessing the quality and value of the basic science underlying—and likely to emerge from —clinical trials will be of considerable value for the foreseeable future. As we go to press, the RAC's future is once again uncertain. In response to pressure from drug companies and some scientists for streamlining the approval process, Dr. Harold Varmus, Director of the NIH, has proposed replacing the RAC with another committee that would be advisory but would not have veto power over standard gene therapy protocols. The role of the FDA would remain as it is.

The political and personal dramas surrounding the attempts to gain RAC and FDA approval for a human trial with the ADA gene have been admirably detailed in Jeffrey Lyons' and Peter Gorner's book *Altered Fates*. Initially, French Anderson had hoped to be able to introduce an ADA gene into hematopoietic stem cells from the bone marrow. Since these stem cells last for the life of an individual, and give rise to all cells of the blood (including the T cells crippled in SCID) correcting the gene defect in stem cells would mean permanent protection from disease. But try as he would, Anderson could never get stable transformation of human bone-marrow stem cells using the retroviral vectors he had generated. The reason for his lack of success is now clear: retroviruses infect only rapidly dividing cells, and it turns out that the vast majority of stem cells from normal bone marrow are not actively dividing at any given time.

Anderson had almost given up when his colleague Michael Blaese suggested another approach; Why not just transform the T cells themselves? If it worked, the effect would only be transient, because T cells do not live very long unless stimulated by foreign antigen. It would probably be necessary to repeat the procedure every few months. But those T cells stimulated by antigen do become long-lived "memory" T cells; in most normal adults, the overwhelming bulk of an immune response is carried by the pool of previously generated memory cells. Over time, Blaese reasoned, a SCID patient in whom even a small proportion of T cells were kept alive long enough to be stimulated by antigen might build up a repertoire of T cells capable of responding to most environmental antigens.

Although initially sceptical, Anderson gradually warmed to the idea. The specific delivery vector proposed by Blaese, Anderson, and their colleague Ken Culver involved a retrovirus that causes leukemia in mice, called MoMLV. Most of the viral genes were removed from the provirus form of MoMLV DNA, and replaced with a ds-cDNA form of an unmutated copy of the human ADA gene. The passenger ADA gene was placed under the control of the retrovirus's own promoter to facilitate transcription into a functional mRNA. This recombinant DNA was then introduced into retroviral packaging cells for conversion to an infectious (but, outside the packaging cells, nonreplicative) retrovirus.

Before submitting an application for the first clinical trials, these recombinant viruses were subjected to a number of intensive laboratory tests. Using T cells isolated from ADA-SCID patients, it was shown that the ADA gene delivered by the retroviral vector could in fact produce ADA in human T cells. Moreover, the resulting enzyme could prevent the buildup of toxic deoxyadenosine, preventing the premature death of the T cells. Next, the vector was used to deliver the ADA gene to the T cells of mice and monkeys, and the altered T cells were then injected into live animals to see if they would continue to function. The results were highly encouraging. Finally, in the late summer of 1990, the RAC and the FDA were sufficiently convinced by the preliminary laboratory data to approve the first human gene therapy trials using the MoMLV-based delivery vector.

Months before, Anderson and other physician-scientists on his team had selected two young girls with ADA-SCID as potential candidates for gene therapy. Ashanti DeSilva, whom we met earlier, would receive the first transfer of the gene. Ashanti was in advanced stages of her disease. Standard therapies, such as PEG-ADA, were not working. Even before final FDA approval had been obtained for the entire gene therapy procedure, samples of T cells were collected from her blood and transfected with the ADA vector in vitro. The cells were first triggered to start dividing, in order to enhance penetration by the retroviral vector. After exposure to the virus, the cells were grown in an incubator for a week or so to expand their total numbers. Final FDA approval was received on the morning of September 14, 1990; that afternoon, four-year-old Ashanti was infused with her own T cells containing the MoMLV-ADA vector, and became the first human being in history to undergo gene therapy for therapeutic purposes. As we know, the procedure went smoothly. After four infusions over a four-month period, Ashi's T cell counts were climbing toward normal. The second young patient to be treated with this procedure, Cynthia Cutshall, received an infusion of her own T cells transformed with the same MoMLV vector on January 31, 1991.*

One of the conditions imposed by the RAC was that these young girls and all subsequent patients receiving ADA gene therapy also be maintained on PEG-ADA. This drug (ADA protein complexed with polyethylene glycol) had been approved by the FDA as a standard treatment for ADA-SCID in 1990, just shortly before the RAC approved ADA gene therapy. In many children it caused a marked initial increase in the number of T cells, alleviating many of the complications of ADA-SCID. On the other hand, some children gain little or no sustainable benefit after a few administrations of the drug, and it is enormously expensive — upwards of $200,000 per year for the average patient.

Because PEG-ADA does not correct the underlying defect, but simply alleviates its symptoms, it must be taken regularly for the life of the patient. Both Ashi and Cynthia were being treated with PEG-ADA at the time they began gene therapy. Although Ashi did not seem to be responding to the drug, it was considered inappropriate to discontinue its use for either patient. Thus evaluation of the efficacy of gene therapy in its first and longest-lasting trial was complicated by the continued administration of a drug whose end effect can be the same as that of the gene therapy: an increase in the number of viable T cells.

Nevertheless, direct analysis of Ashi's T cells has shown that nearly all of them now express the newly inserted ADA gene, and she no longer receives regular infusions of gene-altered T cells. While Cynthia is showing a lower level of expression of the ADA transgene in her T cells, she is definitely using her new gene and is showing a gradual increase in the ability of her T cells to function normally.

Some investigators feel the PEG-ADA may actually be working against

---

*Cynthia was not the second human to be treated by gene therapy; she was actually the fourth. On January 29, 1991, two patients at NIH were treated by gene therapy for an advanced form of cancer. We will examine this aspect of gene therapy in Chapter 8.

the effectiveness of the underlying gene therapy treatment. PEG-ADA helps keep *all* T cells alive, whether or not they have been transduced by the ADA gene. From a gene therapist's point of view, PEG-ADA is helping "bad" (untransduced) as well as "good" T cells (those carrying the ADA gene) to survive. There is reason to believe that, in the absence of PEG-ADA, those good T cells would have a selective advantage for survival, and would eventually outgrow and displace the bad T cells. However, they have been unable to convince the RAC and FDA to allow them to wean these initial patients off the PEG-ADA in order to find out.

That PEG-ADA may indeed be having a less-than-helpful effect for patients undergoing ADA gene therapy is suggested by more recent studies based on French Anderson's original idea of transducing ADA-SCID patients' stem cells rather than T cells. Dr. Donald Kohn, a pediatrician who studied with Michael Blaese at the NIH before joining Children's Hospital in Los Angeles, was presented with an unusual opportunity in early 1993. Three at-risk infants were identified in utero as having ADA-SCID, through a combination of amniocentesis and analysis of their DNA with ADA-specific probes. This is an extraordinary coincidence, given the rarity of the disease. Because of his unique background and training, Kohn was able to convince the RAC to allow him to remove blood from the umbilical cord ("cord blood") from these three infants at birth, and transduce it with the same retroviral ADA vector used for the initial ADA-SCID trials with T cells. The umbilical cord is known to be an unusually rich source of stem cells for the blood cell system; cord blood has actually been used in lieu of bone marrow in certain transplant situations. Moreover, procedures had recently been developed for enriching the concentration of stem cells, taking advantage of a surface molecule on stem cells called CD-34. The RAC agreed to the new trials but insisted that, as in the earlier trials, the infants also receive PEG-ADA as standard therapy. But Kohn was able to convince the RAC to allow him to wean these infants from PEG-ADA.*

This approach appears to be working. Tests carried out shortly after infusion of the altered cord-blood cells showed that about 0.01 to 0.10 percent of the T cells in these infants were expressing the transgene.

---

* Actually, the absolute dose of PEG-ADA was not reduced over time. Rather, as the infants grew, the amount of drug was not increased as their body weight increased, as it normally would be. The result has been an effective reduction in drug dosage.

Although low, these numbers were real and represented the first demonstration that human hematopoietic stem cells can be transduced with a retroviral vector. As the PEG-ADA has been reduced, the overall proportion of T cells expressing the transgene has increased to between one and ten percent—a one hundred-to one thousand-fold increase! Kohn and his colleagues are moving slowly with the PEG-ADA reduction, but are confident their infants will eventually be able to do fine without it. If they are successful, these youngsters (now over four years old) may be the first to achieve the ultimate goal of all gene therapy: a permanent cure of their disease through genetic manipulation alone.

Identification of the Gene for X-linked SCID

As we know, David, the boy in the bubble, was not affected by ADA-SCID, but X-linked SCID. The gene that, when mutated, causes X-linked SCID had not yet been identified during David's lifetime, so gene therapy was never an option for treating him. The biochemical nature of the defect causing X-SCID was not even understood; there was no protein known to be involved that would have allowed working backward to pick up the gene. As recently as 1990 it semed that identification of the X-SCID gene was still a long way off. But the isolation and cloning of this gene was greatly hastened by one of those marvelous situations in which the threads of apparently unconnected inquiries can suddenly entwine in unexpected ways with dramatic consequences.

The pursuit of the X-SCID gene began the hard way, with a detailed study of how the gene segregates in affected families, in order to pin down its chromosomal location as closely as possible. The gross chromosomal association, the X chromosome, was immediately obvious from the fact that this disease affects only males. But further refinements of its location on the X chromosome were slow to emerge because SCID is such a rare disease: there simply were not many families available for study, and individuals affected by the disease do not usually survive very long. Comparison of the inheritance pattern of the X-SCID gene with known X chromosomal markers had narrowed its location to Xq13. But what appears as a dot on a chromosomal map can be millions of nucleotides, much too large a region of DNA to clone and sequence, even if it could be isolated.

While these studies were in progress, other researchers, in what

appeared to be a completely unrelated line of investigation, were busy trying to understand the structure of a molecule found on the surface of T
cells, called the IL-2 receptor (IL-2R). T cells make and release a small
hormonelike molecule called *interleukin-2* (IL-2), which is used by other
cells to help them respond to an infection. Interestingly, T cells themselves use the IL-2 they secrete. During an immune response, T cells
responding to a particular antigenic challenge will release IL-2 into their
immediate vicinity, and then use some of this IL-2 to help them prolif-
erate and produce more of their own kind to fight the infection (see
Figure 4-1). The IL-2 receptor allows them to pick up IL-2 and bring it
inside. (A given T cell can use its own IL-2, or that produced by a neighbor.) T cells also rely heavily on IL-2 during their development in the thymus. As the cells mature, they release IL-2 that they immediately take up
through their IL-2R and use to help them undergo normal cell division.
Without the ability to internalize exogenous IL-2, normal T cell development is aborted shortly after it starts.

The T-cell IL-2 receptor was initially thought to consist of two protein
chains, referred to as IL-2Rα and IL-2Rβ. But certain aspects of IL-2R
function seemed inconsistent with this two-chain model, so researchers
went back for a closer look. A third chain, called IL-2Rγ, was indeed
found. Enough of the Rγ-chain amino acid sequence was determined to
allow synthesis of a nucleic acid probe, which was then used to screen a
cDNA library from a cell line known to be making IL-2Rγ. The corresponding cDNA was isolated and sequenced; the results were published
by a Japanese research team in a 1992 issue of *Science*.

The description and subsequent characterization of the IL-2Rγ chain
explained many of the puzzles relating to IL-2R function. But it remained
for a research team centered at the NIH, which had independently cloned
the IL-2Rγ gene, to make the X-SCID connection. By hybridizing the
gene directly with intact chromosomes, they were able to show that it
bound only to the X chromosome, and specifically to the q13 locus.
Moreover, they showed that DNA from three out of three X-SCID
patients (including a DNA sample preserved from David,) had mutations
in the IL-2Rγ gene; no mutations were found in ten healthy individuals.
These results were confirmed a few months later by a group involved in
the original chromosome mapping studies. Within a very short time it
was clear that the IL-2Rγ gene is the gene that, in mutant form, causes
X-linked SCID.

The knowledge of the nature of the X-SCID protein, gained by study-ing the isolated gene, finally led to an understanding of how the disease is caused (Figure 6-1). As T cells begin to mature in the thymus, they soon reach a point where they need IL-2 to complete their development. In X-SCID children, there is plenty of IL-2 in the thymus, but the emerg-ing T cells are unable to use it because they lack a functional IL-2 recep-tor to bring the IL-2 inside. As a result, these males are born without functional T cells, and hence with virtually no immune protection. The failure to display a fully competent IL-2R on other cells of the immune system further compounds the primary defect.

Through Southern blot tests on small blood samples, portions of the X-SCID gene are already being used as a genetic screening probe to deter-mine which daughters in an X-SCID family are carriers, and whether male fetuses or newborns from at-risk families have inherited a mutant form of the gene. Preclinical experiments with the IL-2γ gene inserted into a retroviral vector have shown that this gene can be delivered to mouse bone-marrow cells, to B cells from X-SCID patients, and to CD-34–enriched umbilical cord cells. Clinical trial protocols involving gene therapy for X-SCID have been submitted for RAC and FDA approval, and may reasonably be expected to get underway sometime in 1997.

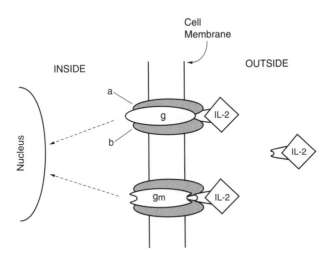

Figure 6-1. The IL-2 receptor and X-linked SCID. The IL-2 receptor, consisting of alpha, beta and gamma subunits, is embedded in the outer membrane of the cell. In the mutant receptor (g_m), IL-2 cannot interact properly with the gamma (g) subunit, and so the appropriate signals are never sent to the nucleus.

7

The Clinical Trials for Cystic Fibrosis

The first gene therapy trials for cystic fibrosis began in the spring of 1993, just over three years after the CFTR gene was cloned and sequenced, and two and a half years after the first ADA-SCID trial. The approach to treating CF by gene therapy is necessarily different from the approach used for ADA-SCID, or any of the other genetic blood-cells diseases ultimately derived from bone marrow. In these latter cases, the cells that are crippled by the genetic defect can be removed from the body, exposed to the gene-bearing vector, and then reimplanted. This form of treatment is referred to as *ex vivo* (or in vitro) gene delivery, with the introduction of the new gene into the target cells occurring outside the body.

Almost all other genetic diseases proposed for treatment by gene therapy will require an in vivo approach; the delivery vector will have to be introduced into the body, as close as possible to the site of the affected tissues and cells, which it must then infect to deliver its passenger gene. It is not practical to inject the vector with its passenger gene into the bloodstream of a patient, and have it somehow find the exact spot in the body where it is needed. Blood travels throughout the body in tightly sealed arteries and veins; this so-called "intravascular space" is almost a separate world within the body. Inducing foreign objects such as viruses or liposomes to exit the bloodstream is difficult enough; their natural tendency is to circulate around the body endlessly until they are finally degraded or have been excreted. Inducing them to cross out of the bloodstream at specific points within the body in a controlled fashion is beyond present technology. So for each disease for which gene therapy is a proposed treatment method, a means must be devised of delivering the vector precisely and efficiently to just those cells that most need the corrected gene.

Since the major site causing illness and death in CF is the respiratory system, the epithelial surfaces of which are readily accessible through the airways, this disease is particularly amenable to in vivo gene therapy. The mucus-producing cells and epithelial cells themselves, into which the delivery vector must carry the CFTR gene, are effectively in direct contact with the outside of the body. Using pressurized atomizers, or by dripping fluid suspensions directly into the bronchioles via the trachea, it is possible to deliver vectors fairly deeply into the lung's passageways. Moreover, the epithelial and mucus-producing cells lining the nose are very similar to those lining the deeper passages, and many experimental procedures designed simply to look at vector safety or transduction efficacy can be done with nasal epithelium, with minimal patient risk or discomfort.

Identification of the Cystic Fibrosis Gene

The identification of the gene responsible for ADA-SCID was, as those things go, relatively straightforward. Like many genes, its isolation was made easier by the fact that the protein had already been at least partially sequenced some years earlier. Identification of the gene for X-SCID was more difficult, but in the end was also greatly accelerated by having protein sequence data to work with. But what is one to do if the protein underlying a disease is completely unknown, let alone isolated and sequenced? How can one go after the gene for a protein one knows absolutely nothing about? Increasingly, as they worked their way through the genes for proteins already sequenced, this was the situation in which molecular biologists found themselves.

The cystic fibrosis gene, CFTR, is a case in point. Nothing was known about the nature of the defective protein in CF, although a great deal of indirect evidence was accumulating that it might be some sort of membrane ion channel. The fact that the protein encoded by this gene was likely to be associated with the cell membrane turned out to be a useful piece of information, but in itself could not guide construction of the all-important DNA probe to isolate the gene.

As with the X-SCID gene, researchers began looking for the CF gene by tracing its pattern of inheritance in families, particularly those with more than one affected child. Using this approach researchers had, over a period of a dozen or so years, traced the CF gene to the long arm of chromosome seven, near band q31 (Figure 7-1). One of the techniques that greatly helped map genes to specific sites on chromosomes is *chromosome banding*, developed at about the same time that somatic cell genetics was beginning to be exploited. For reasons that are not entirely clear, different regions of individual chromosomes interact differently with certain chemical stains, giving rise to very distinct banding patterns. In somatic cell genetic studies, the foreign chromosomes retained in a host cell often fragment, with only a piece of the chromosome being retained. By determining which genes are lost or retained in connection with which bands, genes can be assigned to specific chromosomal regions.

DNA probes already available for the q31 region of chromosome seven had defined two segments of DNA called *MET* and *D7S8*, which were known to lie very close to the CF gene. In virtually every case, a child inheriting a single mutated CF gene from one parent would also inherit that parent's particular allele of MET and D7S8. In genetic parlance, MET, D7S8, and the CF gene were very tightly linked.

The DNA of carrier parents and of their children who had inherited zero, one, or two faulty CF alleles was directly analyzed with these probes to determine the inheritance pattern for MET and D7S8 relative to the CF gene. The results of these kinds of mapping studies strongly suggested that the CF gene would lie somewhere between these two markers. That was the good news; the bad news was that while MET and D7S8 seemed on one level to be intimate neighbors at the q31 locus, they were in fact still separated by somewhere between one and two million base pairs. That is an enormous amount of DNA to analyze. Such analyses are particularly tedious because of the large amounts of "nonsense" DNA present in all animal cells. Nonsense or not, in cases like this all DNA must be sequenced, along with the "real" genes.

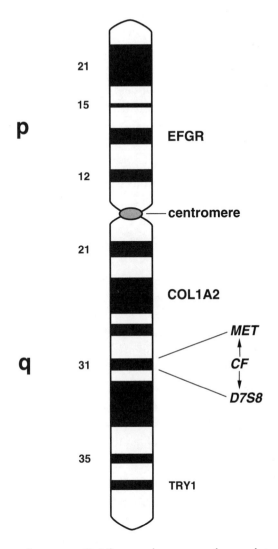

Figure 7-1. Human chromosome 7. Like most chromosomes, human chromosome 7 has two arms of unequal length connected by a centromere. The short arm of each chromosome is referred to as the "p" arm; the long arm is "q". The centromere is where spindle fibers attach in order to segregate the chromosomes into the two daughter cells during mitosis. The banding pattern is not an inherent part of the chromosome; it becomes apparent only after treating the chromosomes with certain stains. However, the banding pattern for each chromosome is the same for each member of the species, and provides useful "landmarks" for gene assignment. The CF gene lies on the long (q) arm of chromosome 7, near band q31. It is flanked by two DNA markers, *MET* and *D7S8*.

Daunting as the task appeared to be, several laboratories led by a major research group in Toronto began the final search at the molecular level for the CF gene. They used a variety of approaches, but most successfully a technique called *chromosome walking*, in which the DNA was sequenced, nucleotide by nucleotide, beginning at the MET and D7S8 markers, and moving from each marker toward the other. This was essentially a brute-force approach, involving dozens of scientists and technicians working over a several-year period. There were at the time only a handful of research groups in the world with the technology, stamina, and funding to undertake such a project. As we will see in later chapters, recent technological advances make such gene hunting much, much easier, but in the mid-1980s it still had to be done the hard way.

Eventually the researchers came across the tell-tale signs of a gene buried in the MET-D7S8 interval. As we know, each gene begins with a "start codon." A number of possible start codons had been spotted among the various cloned fragments from this region, but most of these turned out to be followed fairly shortly by stop codons, suggesting that the start codons were not part of a genuine reading frame. One start codon, however, was followed by a rather long stretch of nucleotides before a stop codon was encountered, and seemed a good candidate for the start site of a real gene. Such stretches of DNA are referred to as *open reading frames* (*ORFs*; pronounced simply "orf"). The putative gene was also preceded by recognizable promoter sequences (see Figure 5-7), which also suggested that the downstream DNA would likely be transcribed into mRNA.

A clever strategy was then used to test further the likelihood that this stretch of DNA actually did contain a gene. DNA fragments containing the ORF were cloned, radiolabeled, and used as probes for Southern blots of DNA libraries of other species. Experience has shown that once nature designs a protein that works well, the plan for that protein tends to become fairly well-conserved in evolution, and widely distributed among species. The amino acid sequence of some proteins may vary by only a few percent between species, although differences of twenty or even thirty percent are more common. Nevertheless, such a high degree of conservation also shows up in the nucleotide sequence of genes, and a gene copy from one species (used as a probe) will often hybridize reasonably well with the homologous DNA of another species. The presence of the same (or slightly modified) sequence in the DNA of several species is usually a good indication that the sequence includes a genuine gene.

The human DNA fragment containing the candidate ORF was found to hybridize rather well with DNA from a number of different species. Other DNA fragments from the MET-D7S8 interval did not hybridize well because "nonsense" DNA sequences by and large are *not* conserved among different species. The ORF-containing DNA was also hybridized with messenger RNA from various human cells to see which cells, if any, appeared to be copying the ORF into mRNA. Messenger RNA tends to be degraded fairly quickly in cells after it is translated; therefore, the mRNA for a specific gene is usually only present when the gene is being actively transcribed. Encouragingly, mRNA complementary to ORF DNA was found mostly in epithelial cells. Finally, the ORF DNA representing a complete CF gene was sequenced in its entirety. The corresponding protein (deduced from the genetic code) turned out to look very much like a membrane protein, which is what had been expected for the CF protein.

Two experimental strategies provided the final proof that the ORF found in the MET-D7S8 interval was the gene which, when defective, causes CF. First, cloning and sequencing of this ORF from CF patients, and comparison of these sequences with the same ORFs from healthy individuals, showed that CF ORFs always had one or more mutations. An analysis of mutants of the CFTR gene has been undertaken by a special international study group called the CF Genetic Analysis Consortium, formed in 1989. Over 300 variants of the CFTR gene have been found in human populations around the world; approximately 230 of these cause mild to severe disease.

The most common mutation (found in over seventy percent of CF patients) was the deletion of an entire codon (three consecutive nucleotides) coding for a single amino acid, phenylalanine, at position 508 in the CF protein, CFTR. This mutation, called ΔF-508, correlated strongly with severe pancreatic dysfunction. Although not causing a frameshift, the resulting protein is severely crippled by a folding defect which prevents it from being properly inserted into the cell membrane. The remaining thirty percent of patients show a total of over 200 different mutations, many of which do involve frameshift mutations (and thus no useable protein), but others of which result in a completed but slightly altered protein with reduced function (Figure 7-2b). This wide range of mutations may help account for the variable clinical symptoms associated with CF. More than one hundred other mutations of the CFTR gene

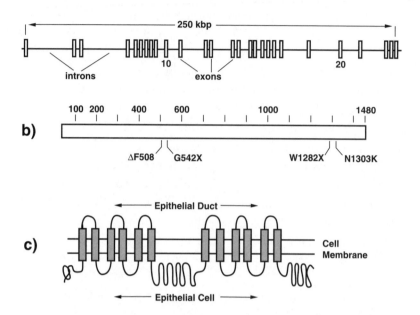

Figure 7-2. The CFTR gene and protein. The CFTR gene (a) is 1480 bp long, and consists of 27 coding exons (boxes), interrupted by 26 introns. Some of the more common other mutations are shown in the linear diagram of the CFTR protein (b). G542X is a point mutation (G toT) in exon 11, which generates a stop codon. W1282X is a similar mutation (G to A) in exon 20. N1303K is a point mutation in exon 21 (C to G) that converts an alanine codon into a lysine codon. (c) The CFTR protein folds back and forth through the cell membrane 12 times. Most of the protein is on the intracellular side of the membrane, and is involved in regulation of CFTR's chloride ion pumping function.

have been detected in people who show no symptoms whatever of CF. These non-disease-causing variants of CFTR presumably have amino acid alterations that are involved in neither the protein's proper folding nor its proper functioning.

The second piece of definitive experimental evidence that CFTR is the defective gene product in CF, involved epithelial cells from CF patients grown outside the body in tissue culture (in vitro).* By the time the CFTR gene was isolated, it was realized that CF epithelial cells were

---

*Most tissues in the body can be dissociated into their component cells, which can then be placed in a bath of nutrients and salts that mimic body fluids ("culture medium"). These cell "cultures" are placed in a warm, moist incubator at body temperature (37° C for mammals), where they can be maintained for days or even months, depending on the cell type.

abnormal in their ability to transport sodium and chloride ions across cell membranes. The ultimate test of the ORF DNA was obviously to determine whether, when a normal version was introduced into CF epithelial cells, it could restore normal sodium and potassium pumping function. Once the corresponding CFTR cDNA was isolated, it was transfected into epithelial cells removed from CF patients and grown in tissue culture. The results left no doubt: when a normal copy of the CFTR gene was introduced into CF cells, and the gene was successfully transcribed and translated into the CFTR protein, CF cells were restored to normal. Cells transformed with mutant forms of the CFTR gene remained abnormal.

Going Clinical

By the time the CFTR gene was isolated, some three dozen gene therapy proocols had been approved by the RAC and the FDA for various human diseases; a dozen or so clinical trials were already underway. There was no doubt in anyone's mind that gene therapy was a major objective of cloning the CFTR gene; research teams around the world began planning strategies for packaging normal forms of the gene into a delivery vector suitable for human gene therapy even before the gene was isolated. Although the protein encoded by CFTR is defective in all cells of a CF patient, and causes serious physiological derangements in a number of organs and tissues, the target of choice for gene therapy is clearly lung and airway tissue. In spite of the fact that the function of organs such as the pancreas, liver, and bowel are seriously compromised in CF, problems in those organs can be handled reasonably well with standard medical treatment. The defects in the lung and airways, on the other hand, still account for the vast majority of untimely deaths from this disease, and all of the protocols submitted so far target airway tissues.

As with ADA-SCID, CF heterozygotes are healthy, which means that a single functional CFTR gene is sufficient for normal operation of a cell. However, it is not clear at the present time exactly which cells in the airway epithelium are critically involved in causing the disease, and thus to which cells the gene must be delivered. The various epithelial linings of the average adult human lung comprise nearly two square meters of surface area, and consist of at least six different cell types, the most common by far being the epithelial cell itself. Other cell types such as the goblet cell, are directly involved in the production of mucus. But in just which of these cells a defective CFTR gene leads to lung disease is still uncertain. Thus the number and density per unit surface area of target cells cannot be precisely estimated. On the other hand, there is every reason to believe that the disease state will be entirely explainable by CFTR defects in some portion of these easily accessible cells. If the gene is delivered to normal cells in the vicinity, no harm will be done.

The obvious viral vector for use in gene therapy of the lungs and airways in CF is adenovirus, since this virus normally seeks out airway tissue and is, by its very nature, adept at entering airway cells. Moreover, it is not a particularly dangerous virus; as many as three-quarters of all children in many urban areas have already been exposed to adenovirus, with no untoward side effects. Retroviral vectors would not be effective in delivering the CFTR gene because the rate of cell division is quite low in epithelial cells. The design of a typical vector used in the initial CF gene therapy trials is shown in Figure 7-3. A form of adenovirus in which several key genes required for viral replication have been removed is cut open, and a ds-cDNA copy of the CFTR gene is inserted. As with retroviral vectors, the crippled vector is then transferred to a packaging cell to grow large amounts of complete, infectious virus.

As with the ADA gene and its retroviral vector, numerous preliminary studies had to be carried out before testing CFTR-adenovirus vectors in humans. First, such vectors were used to infect in vitro epithelial cells isolated from CF patients. The transduced cells rapidly regained the ability to regulate chloride ion transport, showing that the delivery vector could repair human cells. Next, bone-marrow cells were removed from mice and monkeys, infected with the delivery vector, and reinfused back into the animals. Both mice and monkeys were able to produce the human form of CFTR, showing that the vector was able to function in vivo.

Between December 1992 and March 1993, five protocols using replication-deficient adenovirus vectors for Phase I CF gene therapy trials had been submitted to the NIH for consideration. The pathway to RAC and FDA approval had been smoothed somewhat by the ADA-SCID and numerous cancer therapy trials already approved prior to that time. In fact, by the time the cystic fibrosis protocols began to arrive at NIH, the RAC and FDA had approved over a dozen gene therapy trials aimed at curing disease. On April 16, 1993, the first CF protocol received final

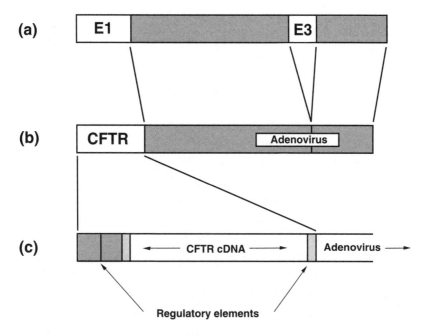

Figure 7-3. A delivery vector for the CFTR gene. a) The adenovirus genome contains two regions (E1 and E3) that are critical to viral replication. These are spliced out using restriction enzymes to create a replication-defective (but still infectious) adenovirus into which a CFTR gene has been inserted where E1 was formerly located (b). The CFTR gene is flanked on either side with regulatory elements (c) that ensure its expression in the targeted cell, and help process its mRNA.

clearance; the next day, a twenty-three year-old man with advanced cystic fibrosis became the first patient ever to be treated with the CFTR gene.

The initial results of this trial, which ultimately involved seven more patients, were reported in September 1994. Like several other Phase I trials, it involved a single administration of the adenoviral-CFTR (AdCFTR) vector to the nasal epithelium and upper airways. About four drops of an AdCFTR saline suspension was administered to the nasal epithelium (on one side only) of each patient. Some patients also received about two-thirds of an ounce of AdCFTR suspension delivered to the bronchi of the lungs through a catheter inserted into a fiber-optic bronchoscope (a device normally used to visually scan the upper airways). The patients were kept under strict isolation before and after the AdCFTR administration, in order to minimize their chances of becoming infected by other environmental pathogens, and of spreading the AdCFTR vector to others.

Cell samples were collected by gently scraping the nose and bronchi at various times after delivery, and the DNA was analyzed for the CTFR gene by Southern blotting. The results of this initial study showed that even at relatively low doses, adenovirus was able to deliver the CFTR gene to both nasal and bronchial epithelium. It is difficult to know precisely what fraction of cells exposed to AdCFTR actually took up the CFTR gene, but estimates are at approximately ten percent. At the very highest dosage used, one patient experienced a transient mild fever that was likely caused by an immune reaction to the crippled virus. However, the fever resolved in a normal fashion, and there were no long-term problems in any of the treated patients. As a result of this reaction the doses proposed for all other clinical trials planned or underway were immediately adjusted downward. As is the rule with Phase I trials, there was no attempt to assess the treatment's impact on the disease itself.

In a subsequent Phase I trial by a different research group, patient immune responses were even more pronounced. Numerous white blood cells were seen infiltrating the nasal epithelium where the viral vector had been deposited. White blood cells mediate inflammation, which can cause local tissue damage, and are the harbingers of the body's concerted immune attack on the invading substance. Possible complications arising from patient immune responses to the delivery vector itself has become one of the major uncertainties about the long-term use of adenovirus for gene therapy—for CF or any other disease.

Adenovirus is a common pathogen in humans, and it is relatively inocuous precisely because the immune system responds so vigorously to adenoviral invasion, promptly clearing the virus from the body before it can cause harm. As noted in Chapter 5, it is relatively easy to disable adenovirus so that it cannot replicate inside human cells, and this is critical for the prevention of disease states associated with uncontrolled pathogen growth. But adenovirus is a rather large virus; even after key genes controlling viral replication have been snipped out, a great many viral genes remain and cannot be practically removed. Upon entry of the replication-deficient adenovirus, these viral genes will begin to direct the synthesis of viral proteins within the target cell, in addition to the human protein encoded by the passenger human gene. The foreign viral proteins within the cell trigger an immune response. The importance of immune resistance in the long-term persistence of adenoviral vectors was highlighted by a nude mouse study in which the vectors survived for many months, compared with a few days to a week in mice with normal immune systems.

Patient immune responses to adenoviral proteins are unlikely in themselves to cause serious harm; because the vector is replication deficient, viral loads will not be large enough to provoke dangerous levels of inflammation. As we have seen, the adenoviral genome (and any passenger genes inserted into it) remains episomal in the host cell nucleus, and production of viral proteins will be transient. But because of this very transience of the response, it seems almost certain that multiple introductions of the vector will be required to achieve clinically significant levels of CFTR protein expression in epithelial cells. Such repeat exposures to even small amounts of viral proteins will drive the immune response to increasing levels of speed and efficiency in dealing with new viruses introduced at each round. Almost certainly, the hyped-up immune response to adenovirus will begin to pick off the virus (and its passenger gene) before it ever reaches its target cells. The immune system, of course, is blameless in all this; it is just doing what millions of years of evolution has selected it to do.

In order to examine possible immunological problems in more detail, the group that organized the initial CF gene therapy trial has obtained RAC and FDA clearance to mount a second Phase I trial involving repeated vector administrations. The first patients were entered into this trial in February 1995. Clearly, from an immunological point of view, the less adenovirus entering the system, the better. To reduce the amount of viral vector needed, scientist members of the gene therapy team reengineered the passenger CFTR gene to make its expression more efficient once inside the cell. The hope is that with more efficient CFTR expression, smaller doses of vector will be needed to produce clinically effective levels of CFTR in cells. At the same time, the scientists removed additional genes from the virus not absolutely essential to its vector function. Bronchial swipes will be taken monthly from patients to determine whether and to what extent the CFTR gene is being expressed in bronchial cells. The level of the patient immune response to adenovirus will be carefully monitored as a function of the number and strength of vector doses administered. As with the original Phase I trial, the impact of treatment on the patients' disease state will not be monitored, since that is not the objective of the trial. However, the ultimate question will be whether enough CFTR genes can be introduced into enough epithelial cells to have a likely impact on disease before the immune system begins to interfere with vector delivery. That will be determined in a subsequent Phase II trial if the results of the current study are sufficiently encouraging.

Alternate Delivery Vectors

As the immunological problems associated with adenovirus as a delivery vector became increasingly apparent, several clinical research groups across the country began experimenting with liposomes for CFTR-gene delivery. As discussed in Chapter 5, liposomes are synthetic lipid (fat) vesicles that can be used to package and deliver within the body a wide range of pharmacological reagents, including DNA. Two groups have incorporated the CFTR gene into liposomes, and are using them for Phase I trials in humans. First, the CFTR gene is incorporated into a standard bacterial plasmid containing the information necessary for DNA replication once it enters a mammalian cell. As with adenovirus vectors, DNA introduced into cells via liposomes remains episomal. These liposomes were first tested on epithelial cells from CF patients in vivo, and on airway passages of mice and rats in vivo. Uptake and expression of the CFTR gene was verified in both types of study.

The initial human trials have restricted delivery of the liposomes to the nasal epithelium, since cells can readily be recovered from this site to determine whether the DNA has been taken up by the epithelial cells, and whether it has directed the synthesis of functional CFTR protein. The first results to be published from such a study showed that the liposomes caused no harm to patient tissues per se, and did not induce a measurable immune response. This study involved fifteen male CF patients, all with the ΔF508 mutation to insure comparability of results. Nine of the patients received the CFTR gene in liposomes; six others were treated with empty liposomes as a control. The liposome suspension was dripped directly onto the nasal epithelium. Small biopsies were taken from the treatment area four days later and examined for the presence of the gene and for infiltrating white blood cells. Gene expression was seen in all but one of the patients receiving it; white-cell infiltration was minimal.

Treated nasal tissue was also examined for its ability to transport sodium and chloride ions, a measure of CFTR protein function. Positive responses were seen in most of the patients receiving the gene, in one case reaching twenty percent of the levels of CFTR function seen in healthy individuals. Given that this was only a Phase I trial to test safety and not efficacy, the results are encouraging. As expected, CFTR function was transient, peaking in a few days and disappearing after a week, reflecting the episomal nature of the DNA delivered and highlighting the need for repeated administrations.

Given the transient nature of CFTR gene expression in these early trials, the patients obviously experienced no meaningful improvement in their disease. Again, that is not the point of a Phase I trial. But in this first use of liposomes for gene therapy, clear evidence was obtained that liposomes bypass many of the problems experienced with viral vectors, and that liposomes can indeed be used to deliver genes to airway tissue. Great effort is now being devoted to making liposome delivery more efficient.

Clearly there are many challenges to be met in terms of delivering CFTR genes to the right tissues and getting them into the cells that need them. Also, stabilizing gene expression in transduced cells or devising means for periodic readministration of new genes without provoking a host immune response are concerns. While we should not underestimate the magnitude of the challenges that remain, these may well be largely technical. The difficulties encountered so far with CF gene therapy are no greater than those that plagued the beginnings of other major medical advances. It seems unlikely that these problems represent a more fundamental resistance of the body to genetic manipulation, as some have claimed. Both immunization and organ transplantation seemed in their own times unnatural manipulations of the body that could not be tolerated; time has proven otherwise.

8

Gene Therapy for Monogenic Disorders

What Have We Learned, and Where Are We Going?

When we take into account all of the diseases caused by external agents such as infectious microorganisms, we are still left with a rather large array of human disorders arising from internal dysfunctions. It is now clear that a significant proportion of these *idiopathic* diseases are caused by defective genes, nearly all of which are inherited. Some of these diseases, such as SCID and CF, are monogenic, while others (diabetes, for example) are polygenic, involving several genes at once. The possibility of treating monogenic disorders by introducing into crippled cells a functional copy of the underlying gene was one of the first benefits perceived for the application of molecular biology to human medicine. Applications for treating diseases such as cancer and AIDS followed soon thereafter. The possibility that gene therapy could be of use in treating polygenic diseases is at present remote; the likelihood of getting multiple genes into affected cells and having them expressed in a coordinated and well-regulated fashion is beyond present technology.

So far we have taken a close look at two inherited monogenic diseases that are potentially amenable to gene therapy. ADA-SCID is a good model for monogenic blood cell disorders generally; CF is more typical of hereditary diseases affecting the rest of the body's cells and tissues. The number of genes associated with human monogenic hereditary disorders that have now been isolated and cloned for study continues to grow, although the rate at which such genes are being discovered has slowed temporarily. Retrieving copies of complete genes from genomic DNA, which is essential to a full understanding of how a particular gene works, now takes only a matter of weeks or perhaps a few months; the time-consuming and costly methods used to prise the CFTR gene out of the human genome are a thing of the past. Very shortly after the turn of the century, thanks to something called the Human Genome Project, *every* human gene, in its complete genomic form, should be available to any laboratory that wants to study it, or consider it for use in gene therapy.

In addition to cystic fibrosis and ADA-SCID, gene therapy clinical trials are now underway for at least half a dozen other single-gene hereditary diseases (Table 8-1), and preclinical studies for a dozen or so more diseases are nearing completion. Following is a brief sampling of progress in some of these trials and studies:

Table 8-1. *Some common single-gene hereditary diseases.*

(The human gene responsible for each of these diseases has been identified and cloned. Clinical trials have already begun for those marked with an asterisk, and should begin in the near future for those marked with a pound sign. Preclinical studies for the remaining diseases are nearing completion.)

ADA-SCID*	Huntington's disease
Bruton's agammaglobulinemia[#]	Lesch-Nyhan disease[#]
Chronic granulomatous disease*	Lou Gehrig's disease
Cystic fibrosis*	Neurofibromatosis
Duchenne muscular dystrophy	Purine nucleoside phosphorylase deficiency*
Familial hypercholesterolemia*	Sickle cell anemia
Fanconi's anemia*	Tay-Sach's disease
Gaucher's disease*	Thalassemia
Hurler's syndrome[#]	X-linked SCID[#]
Hunter's syndrome*	

Rheumatoid arthritis (RA) is a painful, debilitating autoimmune disease characterized by rampant inflammation of the joints. It is ordinarily controlled by systemic (through the bloodstream) administration of anti-inflammatory agents, and occasionally by injection of such drugs—some of which are proteins—directly into the joints. But these agents, especially when administered systemically, often interfere with the body's normal immune responsiveness, which restricts the amount that can be administered and limits the agents' usefulness. In a recent NIH preclinical study, cells taken directly from the joints of rats with arthritis were transduced in vitro with a retrovirally packaged human gene encoding a potent anti-inflammatory protein. The transduced cells were then injected back into the inflamed joints, and the subsequent progress of the disease monitored. Rats treated with this form of gene therapy experienced greatly reduced swelling of joints, and less inflammatory destruction of local tissue. The investigators concluded that the anti-inflammatory protein was 10,000 times more effective when administered by this form of gene therapy than when administered systemically. There was no effect on any other tissues in the body, and normal immune responses were not compromised. Clinical trials in humans are planned for the near future.

Cardiovascular disease. Arteries clogged by cholesterol and other debris can cause fatal heart attacks when the arteries are in the heart itself. But they can also cause serious problems elsewhere in the body. Blockages in major arteries cause thousands of Americans each year to lose limbs to gangrene and subsequent amputation. In the heart, bypass surgery or balloon angioplasty is often effective, but such techniques have been only marginally effective in limbs. It turns out that the body makes a protein, vascular endothelial growth factor (VEGF), that stimulates the production of new blood vessels. In a recent clinical trial at Tufts University in Boston, doctors introduced the gene for VEGF into the muscle tissue surrounding a blocked artery in the leg of a woman who had an advanced case of gangrene. (This is an example of single-gene enhancement therapy, rather than gene replacement.) The patient experienced an eighty-percent increase in blood flow to the affected leg.

Unfortunately, the gangrene was too advanced, and the woman still lost the leg to amputation. But permission has now been granted to extend the procedure to patients with less-advanced disease. Interestingly, in this procedure "naked DNA" was used; the gene (without a vector) was simply smeared onto the surface of a balloon similar to that used for angioplasty. The balloon was then inserted into the blocked artery and inflated, pressing the DNA into the surrounding wall, which then developed new (unclogged) arterial branches that penetrated surrounding tissues. It was learned that the cells comprising blood vessels will take up DNA relatively efficiently without the aid of a delivery vector. The lack of a requirement for a delivery vector circumvents completely questions of safety; the results so far suggest this approach may become a very important adjunct to managing the circulatory complications of hypercholesterolemia.

Familial Hypercholesterolemia. One subset of patients suffering from blocked arteries are those with the inherited monogenic disorder, familial hypercholesterolemia. These individuals have two defective copies of the gene encoding the low-density lipoprotein (LDL) receptor, which helps remove excess cholesterol from the blood. When this receptor is missing in the body, dangerously high cholesterol levels are present in the blood. This condition is difficult to treat, and affected individuals experience debilitating or lethal cardiovascular problems very early in life. One of the main action sites of the LDL receptor is at the surface of liver cells. In recent clinical trials involving five patients aged seven to forty-one years, a small portion of liver was removed, from which single liver-cell suspensions were prepared. These were then transduced in vitro with a retroviral vector containing the LDL-receptor gene, and infused back into the patients' livers. All patients have shown significantly reduced levels of serum cholesterol as a result.

Hurler Syndrome. Hurler syndrome is a devastating inherited disorder that results in gross skeletal abnormalities in children, most notably in the head and neck region. There are also gross distortions of internal structures, and these children usually live at most a half dozen or so years, dying from respiratory or cardiac failure. This recessive disorder is caused by the lack of a single enzyme, α-L-iduronidase. Although this enzyme is absent in all cells of the body, like ADA deficiency the key cells causing most of the symptoms are bone-marrow derived — in this case macrophages rather than T cells. Very recently, the gene for α-L-iduronidase has been introduced into human CD-34⁺ stem cells; the macrophages deriving from these stem cells were completely normal. Clinical trials for correcting Hurler syndrome in affected infants should begin shortly.

Potential strategies for treating a number of other monogenic disorders, such as the inherited form of amyelotrophic lateral sclerosis (ALS or "Lou Gehrig's disease"), are currently in the planning stages. Yet none of the patients involved in any of the studies carried out so far has been cured of their disease. So why do we keep adding new diseases to the list of those to be treated by gene therapy? What, if anything, has been accomplished so far, and where is all this taking us?

The major driving force behind gene therapy is a compelling underlying logic. Genes are no longer a mystery. They are stretches of DNA that dictate the primary structure of proteins. They are flanked by other stretches of DNA that regulate their expression in cells. We know how genes work, and why they sometimes fail. The technology to isolate genes from human DNA, grow these genes in suitable vectors, and reintroduce them into human cells is now essentially routine. These surrogate genes function perfectly normally in their new cellular environment, particularly if they are inserted into the host cell DNA. We know enough now about the regulation of gene expression to ensure that a surrogate gene can respond to normal regulatory signals in its new environment, making the corresponding protein in the right amounts at the right times. Years of experience working with cells and genes in vitro tells us that it absolutely is possible to repair genetic defects by gene replacement.

Yet it is also absolutely true that gene therapy in the clinic has so far had very little impact on human disease. What is the compelling logic in pursuing a course of treatment that has failed hundreds of times over? First of all, as we know, none of the trials mounted so far were *intended* to cure patients, or even to relieve their symptoms. The Phase I trials currently in progress are simply part of the process of moving any new procedure or therapeutic agent from the laboratory to the clinic. In each of these cases, experiments carried out in basic research laboratories had shown that a normal copy of a gene introduced into a cell bearing mutant copies of that gene could be "cured" of the problems caused by the mutant gene. Evidence was also obtained that gene transfer could work in vivo, using either an animal model or human tissues implanted into a nude mouse. This kind of data provides a sound rationale for using the procedure in human patients, but at some point someone has to take the first step; at some point the experiments (and they are still that) must be transferred into live human beings. No one does this lightly, and it is done in carefully controlled stages. The very first human exposure to a new drug or procedure in a Phase I trial has intentionally limited goals: to test the safety of that drug or procedure in a human body, to be certain that the data gathered in preclinical laboratory tests have a reasonable chance of being reproduced in human patients, and to find out what difficulties might be encountered in a real-life clinical setting. A Phase I clinical trial is thus very much like the early rounds of a boxing match, with the opponents sparring, jabbing, feinting, weaving, and searching out one another's strengths and weaknesses.

What we have learned from gene therapy clinical trials so far is that genes prepared in the laboratory *can* be introduced into human cells, either in vivo or in vitro, and that the transferred genes *can* function in their new surroundings for periods of weeks to years. Importantly, all of the data collected so far suggest that gene therapy as currently practiced is safe. Larger numbers of patients, treated over many more years, will be required to confirm this absolutely, but none of the 500 or so patients treated through mid-1996 (some of whom are now five years into treatment) have suffered more than mild and transient side effects; the vast majority have suffered no ill effects at all. The available evidence also suggests that the transferred genes function in a manner indistinguishable from their counterparts in normal human cells. Thus there is good reason to believe that if enough genes can be transferred into enough cells, and if their expression can be maintained over a long enough period of time, gene therapy will be able to correct the underlying defect for a great many diseases.

The most impressive results to date have been obtained with some of the children treated with the ADA-SCID gene. These first patients are still showing strong expression of the transferred genes five years after treatment. One of these young patients has likely been cured of her disease by gene therapy, although this cannot yet be stated unequivocally. (The patient is still maintained on PEG-ADA, and will be for the foreseeable future, though nearly everyone agrees that this case proves that gene therapy *can work in humans*.) The follow-up trials with other SCID children look very promising, and it now seems certain that gene therapy will have a major impact on monogenic blood-cell diseases. The fact that the cells to be treated can be removed from the body, transfected with a retroviral vector, and tested for expression of the passenger gene before being returned to the body is a great advantage. The cells can be exposed to an enormous excess of delivery vector, increasing the chances that a reasonable proportion of them will be transduced. Once transformed with a retrovirally packaged gene, a blood cell will carry that gene as part of its own DNA for the rest of its life.

For diseases such as ADA-SCID, the target of choice for the retroviral vector and its passenger gene would be the blood stem cells, which in adults reside in the bone marrow. The cells produced from stem cells, such as T cells, B cells, and macrophages, have relatively short lifespans, meaning that transduction of these mature cell forms would have to be repeated over and over as they die off and are replaced by new stem-cell progeny. Stem cells, on the other hand, last a very long time, perhaps indefinitely; transduction would have to take place only once to ensure a lifetime supply of transduced progeny. Unfortunately, bone-marrow stem cells divide only rarely, and a limitation of retroviruses, as we have seen, is the fact that most of them can only transduce actively dividing cells. The reason for this is that in most cases the retroviral DNA can only enter the nucleus (and thus gain access to the host DNA) when the nuclear membrane dissolves temporarily at the time of cell division. With present levels of efficiency of retroviral transduction of nondividing cells, it has been virtually impossible to achieve significant levels of gene delivery to mature human bone-marrow stem cells. Interestingly, mouse stem-cell transduction with retroviruses is very efficient, leading researchers to believe the same may well be true of human stem cells, if we could just find the right retroviral vector. Some of the techniques used with the mouse cells have been applied to monkey bone-marrow cells with encouraging signs of success. It seems highly likely that a close study of the differences among the mouse, monkey, and human systems should result in the development of a useable means for retroviral transduction of human bone-marrow stem cells in the near future.

Human umbilical cord-blood stem cells, on the other hand, do seem to be more susceptible to retroviral transduction, for reasons that are not clear at present. One strategy that seems promising for both bone marrow and cord blood is to treat them just prior to exposure to retrovirus with chemical signals (*cytokines*) that the body uses to bring cells from a resting state into active cell division. This normally happens whenever the supply of stem-cell-derived blood cells falls too low in the circulation. These cytokines are well known to researchers, and seem to greatly increase the efficiency of human stem-cell transduction. Several children have been treated using this approach, and the results are highly promising.

An even more imaginative approach may be to use HIV as a gene-delivery vector. HIV is unique among retroviruses in being equipped with a special mechanism for getting its proviral DNA into the nucleus of cells, whether they are dividing or not. With a properly engineered HIV genome, it could be possible to deliver genes safely and stably into the DNA of any target cell, not just cells that divide. However, there are two problems with HIV. The first, of course, is the terrible disease it can cause, though, once disabled by removing key genes needed for replication, HIV is just another replication-deficient virus. The safety of such viruses has been proved beyond any shadow of a doubt. With such a deadly virus, safety procedures may have to be made even more stringent than usual, as much for political as for scientific reasons. But the fear that attends using something as deadly as HIV for routine gene therapy, even in disabled form, may also be overcome by using other viruses in the HIV family (*lentiviruses*), such as the feline or bovine immunodeficiency viruses. These viruses, which are not pathogenic in humans, also possess the ability to penetrate a nondividing nucleus.

A second problem with HIV as a delivery vector is that, unlike other retroviruses, it has a very narrow target-cell range. Whereas most retroviruses will readily infect a large number of different cell types, HIV (at least in humans, which is not this virus' normal host) readily infects only cells displaying the CD4 surface molecule. It does this by using a special molecule called gp120 that is part of its outer protein coat (gp is an abbreviation for glycoprotein; 120 refers to its atomic unit size). The gp 120 molecule specifically recognizes and binds to target cells' CD4. One solution would be to genetically engineer the part of gp120 that binds CD4 so that it binds to molecules more widely distributed on cell surfaces. Such alterations are fairly straightforward and could be tailored to specific needs. For example, in cases where the object is to deliver a potentially harmful gene to a cell (e.g., in cancer treatments), it may be desirable to restrict rather than enlarge the range of cells with which the delivery vector interacts.

Researchers have recently found that by removing the HIV genes that code for the coat proteins, and replacing them with the corresponding genes from a virus that can infect nerve tissue (but which is not itself a retrovirus), HIV could be used to deliver genes to brain cells, which never divide once an organism has reached maturity. This very direct demonstration of HIV's potential for gene therapy of nondividing cells is a tremendous step forward.

All in all, the future for gene therapy in the treatment of monogenic blood disorders such as ADA-SCID and even Hurler's syndrome looks very bright indeed. Solving the problem of getting genes into human stem cells is almost certainly just a matter of time. Unfortunately, in the larger framework of human disease, these blood-cell-based disorders are barely the tip of the iceberg. Conditions such as cystic fibrosis are much more representative of the panoply of monogenic diseases that plague us, and also underscore some of the challenges that must be met if gene therapy is to become an effective form of medical treatment. The major problem encountered so far is the relatively low efficiency of delivery of therapeutic genes to cells in vivo. Part of this is due to the fact that it is difficult to achieve high ratios of vector to target cells in vivo. Blood cells can be literally bathed in vector for long periods of time during transduction in vitro. In vivo, excess vector is quickly washed away by extracellular fluids. This could presumably be overcome by repeat administrations of vector but, as we have seen, many viral delivery vectors cause a gradual buildup of host immune defenses that neutralize subsequent deliveries. Although researchers are working to reduce the immunogenicity of viral vectors, it seems unlikely that large and complex viruses such as adenovirus could ever be made completely invisible to the immune system, especially if life-long repeat administrations must be given.

Retroviruses are much less immunogenic, but have not been used for gene delivery in vivo because very few cells are actively dividing in vivo. One way around this problem could be to use a suitably engineered retrovirus, with a capacity for nuclear penetration, for in vivo gene delivery. Retroviruses are extremely small, and provoke much less of an immune response. Moreover, since the gene delivered by a retrovirus becomes permanently embedded in the host cell's DNA, repeat administrations would not have to be open-ended; once a critical number of cells are transduced, treatment could be stopped.

In the end, the best gene delivery vectors may not be viruses at all. We have seen that DNA can also be delivered to cells in liposomes, lipid bodies with many properties of cell membranes. There are already clinical trials underway using liposomes to deliver the CFTR gene to CF patients.

The problem to date with liposomes has been the low efficiency of DNA delivery in vivo. One of the great advantages of viruses is that they have receptors (such as the gp120 molecule of HIV) that allow them to bind with high efficiency to target cells. Considerable attention is currently being devoted to developing liposomes that have specific cell-targeting molecules such as gp120 engineered onto their surface. Another approach is to trap retroviruses into liposomes, creating a so-called "virosome"; recent studies showed that the combination of the two increases the efficiency of retroviral transduction up to fifty-fold.

It may even be possible in some cases to hook a targeting molecule right onto the DNA itself, bypassing the need for a delivery vector altogether. Viruses also have other "tricks" that they use to protect and properly route DNA once it has been taken up by the cell. Scientists are studying how some of this viral information could be included with inert DNA particles to further increase efficiency of transduction. Of particular interest would be the mechanism used by retroviruses to stably integrate the DNA into the host-cell genome. What we may very well eventually see is an "artificial virus," perhaps wrapped in a liposome, that has many of the advantages of an intact virus for getting DNA into cells, without any of the disadvantages in terms of safety or immunogenicity. Enormous energy and creativity is being poured into the problem of delivering DNA to cells in vivo in amounts large enough to correct underlying genetic defects. It seems certain that this problem will be solved in the next few years.

But there is nevertheless a strong sense at present that it may be time to step aside and digest what has taken place in gene therapy thus far, and address at a basic research level some of the technical problems that have arisen with nonblood-cell gene delivery, before rushing ahead with new clinical trials involving additional genes. DNA delivery systems now in the laboratory are much more efficient than those used in clinical trials presently underway, but they could almost certainly be made even *more* efficient. Rather than rush the current generation of new delivery systems to the clinic, why not sit back for a year or two and wait for the next wave of improvements? Scientists are also tinkering with better ways to stabilize genes once they have been successfully introduced into cells, and better ways to regulate their expression. The rate of progress in the laboratory is so impressive that it would seem premature to try to cash in on what is state of the art today, since the art will almost certainly be even more impressive a year or two from now.

Thus, while in the long run we may expect to see many more human disease genes made available for clinical trials, in the short run, there may seem to be little progress. Of the fifty most recent clinical trials reviewed by the RAC and FDA, in fact only three were proposed for monogenic diseases; the rest involved either cancer or AIDS. There are several reasons for this. The number of human genes that have been cloned and definitely associated with monogenic disorders, although growing rapidly, is at the moment still rather limited. Very few—if any—laboratories are pursuing the isolation and cloning of disease genes on an ad hoc basis. The Human Genome Project will eventually uncover *all* such genes in a systematic fashion, but even after they have been identified, several years of intense laboratory study will be required before any disease gene is ready for use in clinical trials. For each gene we will need to understand how it is expressed in living cells, and how this expression is normally regulated. Also, a suitable delivery vector system will have to be developed for each gene, and its effectiveness in vitro and in vivo established.

A second reason that gene therapy for monogenic disorders has been at least temporarily eclipsed by clinical trials for cancer and AIDS is that the number of patients involved in all but a few monogenic diseases (cystic fibrosis is one obvious exception) is small, and there is presently very little private sector financial support for research into these diseases. This is of course not a problem unique to gene therapy; it is equally true for research into the development of other forms of treatment for both genetic and nongenetic diseases. The patient base in cancer and AIDS on the other hand is quite large, and there is a reasonable expectation that a company committing resources to gene-based therapies for these diseases would have a chance of recovering its investment. The genes involved in treating these diseases, and the strategies for using them, are also largely already in hand. Increasingly, we see the financial support for research and clinical trials for cancer and AIDS coming from private drug and pharmaceutical companies, whereas research into gene therapy for monogenic disorders continues to be funded almost entirely by the federal government. Once the costs of developing a reasonable treatment protocol (by far the largest expense for any new treatment or drug) have been underwritten by the government, of course, the private sector will usually participate in bringing the treatment to market with standard manufacturing and marketing techniques.

In the beginning, gene therapy was attended by a good deal of hope, and a great deal of hype. Like any other group of human beings, scientists and physicians have among them their share of carnival barkers and hand-wringers, fanatical optimists and unpersuadable pessimists. But almost every major advance in modern medicine—vaccination, antibiotics, organ transplantation—has passed through exactly the same sequence of events before assuming its place as part of the standard medical armamentarium. Gene therapy is barely five years old; it doesn't work perfectly yet, but the compelling logic that drives it, and the ingenuity and resourcefulness of those committed to its success augur extremely well for the future. As Theodore Friedmann said in a recent *Nature Medicine* commentary:

> Human gene therapy has not yet come of age, but there is no justification for doubting its eventual success as an adjunct to traditional therapies or as a definitive therapy on its own. The most revolutionary aspect of human gene therapy has been the conceptual one, and that phase is over. We have now reached the difficult evolutionary stage of making it work. . . . The waves of enthusiasm and caution, even mania and depression, that accompany our first steps to implement the concept of human gene therapy should not be seen as an indication the effort has failed or that it is unworthy.

9

Gene Therapy for Cancer

Just two decades ago, our thinking about cancer, and especially its treatment, was as fragmented as the disease itself appeared to be. Oncologists were a frustrated lot. There seemed to be as many different diseases called cancer as there were different cells in the body; any one of them could become cancerous, and each of the resulting diseases seemed to require a completely different treatment approach. The treatments developed during these decades were still based on a view of cancer cells as some sort of biological renegades, crazy and dangerous cells that had to be destroyed at all costs. Powerful weapons based on radiation and chemotherapy were developed as adjuncts to the surgeon's knife. A few cancers did in fact succumb to this approach, but not many; to this day, half of all cancers remain essentially untreatable.

Our thinking about cancer has changed remarkably in recent years. Bone cancer still looks different from brain cancer; skin cancer is still treated differently than lung cancer. But the current focus is on understanding what *causes* cancer in the first place, and here the emphasis is on what cancers have in common, rather than on what makes them different. Cancer can be caused by external agents—radiation, chemicals, certain viruses—or by mistakes made within a cell, usually in connection with DNA replication. And indeed, any cell or tissue in the body *can* give rise to a tumor. But ultimately *every cancer is a disorder of DNA*. The processes by which a normal cell is converted into a tumor cell (*oncogenesis*) are in most cases extraordinarily subtle and complex. Yet all cancer cells share a single, common feature: they have their lost ability to regulate DNA synthesis and cell division. And the regulatory elements governing these processes lie in the DNA itself, in our genes.

All multicellular animals that reproduce sexually begin life as a single cell (a zygote) formed by the union of two germ cells, a sperm and an ovum in humans. The stages of development immediately following zygote formation are characterized by extraordinarily rapid and uniform cell division (mitosis). In many ways the developing organism is very much like a small tumor, at least initially. All of the embryonic cells arising through mitosis inherit a set of chromosomes identical to those in the cell from which they are derived; genetically, the cells in our bodies are basically clones of the original zygote from which we came. The fact that the cells comprising an adult organism appear to be so different from one another (and from the zygote) is a consequence of differential gene expression over developmental time.

As embryological development proceeds, the process of unbridled cell division is gradually brought under control, and at this point any similarity with a tumor ends. True, some cells continue to divide until the body reaches its final size and shape. Even in the fully formed individual, many cells retain the potential to divide if called upon in an emergency —wound-healing, for example. A few cells, most notably those giving rise to the various cells of the blood system, continue vigorous cell division throughout life. But the story of fetal, embryological, and childhood development is one of a continual reining in of cellular proliferation, and of bringing growth processes increasingly under the most stringent regulation. The operation of something as complex as the human body requires delicate coordination and precise control of every single cell comprising an individual. All of the parts of the body must work together, and indeed physically fit together, within very strict limits; if the cells of any given tissue enter into "inappropriate" cell division at the wrong time or in the wrong place and invade each other's territory, the results can be disastrous. If not immediately removed by the immune system, or otherwise brought under control, these undisciplined cells can give rise to the disease we call cancer.

Aside from a few strongly hereditary cancers, it is not generally the case that a single gene stands between us and cancer. In this sense, cancer is very different from SCID and CF. Cancer tends to develop fairly late in life because in most cases more than one gene must be lost or mutated for a cancer to develop. The threat of cells breaking free of the controls placed on inappropriate cell division is so great that there are multiple security systems in place to be sure it does not happen. The multigenic nature of cancer means that the standard approach to gene therapy, augmentation of a single defective gene with a normal copy of that gene, will in many cases not be useful.

There is another fundamental difference between cancer and genetic diseases such as CF or SCID that is important to remember. In diseases caused by a single gene defect that results in abnormal cell function, the object is to transduce as many affected cells as possible with the transgene, but transduction of every single affected cell (which is, in some cases, every cell in the body) is neither possible nor necessary to achieve an acceptable result. In ADA-SCID, for example, it seems clear that even a small number of transduced stem cells, or transduced mature T cells, will have a selective survival advantage over nontransduced cells and will eventually displace defective cells in the immune system. Even in a disease such as CF, where transduced epithelial cells will most likely *not* have a significant survival advantage over nontransduced cells, rescue of only a portion of the cells may well be sufficient to stimulate the production of enough normal mucus to achieve measurable amelioration of disease. In all "standard" gene therapy, the object is to stably transduce a reasonable proportion of cells and restore them to near-normal function for as long as possible.

In treating cancer, we have exactly the opposite situation. The purpose of placing a transgene inside a cancer cell is either to kill the cell, or else to restore it to normal—to retard its wild and unregulated growth. Thus the survival advantage will always be to the *untreated* cells in cancer gene therapy. Anything that inhibits only some of the tumor cells simply makes more room for the remaining cells, which keep on growing. What that means at the practical level is that somehow every single tumor cell must ultimately be brought under control by a given treatment, or that treatment will not work: the surviving cancer cells will simply grow back. This is a formidable hurdle to overcome, even for molecular medicine.

There are, nevertheless, a number of approaches to treating cancer based on the general principles of molecular medicine that are highly promising. In fact, of the more than one hundred gene therapy trials currently approved by federal regulatory agencies, over half are for the treatment of cancer. Of the fifty most recently reviewed (not all are yet approved), forty are cancer-related. For the small number of cancers in which a single defective gene seems to be a major cause of the problem (probably not more than ten percent of all cancers), standard gene replacement therapies such as those developed for CF or ADA-SCID may be useful. The object of this approach is not to kill the tumor cell, but to try to coax it back onto a pathway of regulated growth and development. For those tumors for which gene replacement will not be useful, we can try to overcome the tumor by fine-tuning the body's own responses to oncologic disease. Rather than trying to destroy a tumor directly with radiation or chemical poisons, we can attempt to make it more readily visible to the body's own immune system in an approach called "adoptive immunotherapy." Finally, if gene replacement and adoptive immunotherapy are inappropriate, and we must rely on more traditional radiation or chemotherapy therapies, we can use molecular medicine to make cancer cells more sensitive to these treatments so that the body generally doesn't have to suffer the horrendous side effects of all-out, maximal-force attacks on the tumor. Each of these approaches to treating cancer is already the subject of federally approved clinical trials. We will examine a few typical examples in the following sections.

The Genes Involved in Cancer

Cells most often lose control of DNA replication and cell division through mutation or loss of the genes that keep these processes tightly regulated in normal cells. We have learned a great deal about these genes, and how they carry out their tasks, in the last dozen years. In a small number of cases, mutations in a single gene controlling cell division can strongly predispose to the development of cancer. There are two major categories of such "strong" cancer-causing genes. The first category consists of *oncogenes*, whose normal protein products are involved in telling a resting cell when to divide.* Ordinarily this only comes about in response to a signal arriving at the cell surface from somewhere else in the body, telling the cell it is alright to start dividing. When this external signal is withdrawn, the oncogenes that are involved in the proper reading and processing of these signals turn off, and the cell promptly returns to the resting state. Certain mutations in a single allele of an oncogene may activate the oncogene (or the protein it encodes) in the absence of normally required signals. The result is unscheduled cell division and formation of a tumor. More than fifty oncogenes have been defined in humans, and they are detectable in a large proportion of human cancers. Oncogene-induced tumors can only arise spontaneoulsy during the lifetime of an individual; oncogenes cannot be transmitted through the germline. If an oncogene were passed through the germ cells to an embryo, every cell in that embryo would have a major problem regulating cell division. The result would almost certainly be massive fetal abnormalities and spontaneous abortion. And in fact, no hereditary cancer has ever been traced to a mutant oncogene.

The second category of genes involved in cancer are the *tumor-suppressor genes*. These genes regulate the cell's internal machinery for suppressing cell division, and make sure it stays in the "off" state when cell division is not needed. Tumor suppressor genes and their protein products provide a major defense against the unscheduled cell division that may result from an oncogene mutation. Tumor suppressor genes are also involved in repairing damaged DNA. In order for a tumor to develop as a result of a faulty tumor-suppressor gene, *both* alleles of the gene must be defective, since in this case the gene product is involved in turning off proliferation. As with most genes, a single normal allele is sufficient to carry out the active function of the gene — in this case, suppression of cell division. One faulty allele would be insufficient to cause cancer; the second allele would produce more than enough of the protein keep cell division under control.

Tumor-suppressor genes can be involved in strongly hereditary cancers

---

*The term oncogene formally refers only to the mutated form of the corresponding normal gene involved in initiation of cell division. The normal form of the gene is referred to as a *proto-oncogene*. However, for simplicity's sake, we will use the term oncogene to refer to both forms of the gene.

through a mechanism called "loss of heterozygosity." What is inherited is a single faulty allele of the particular suppressor gene. Inheritance of two faulty alleles is unlikely; it would be the equivalent of inheriting a single mutated oncogene, and would cause serious problems for the developing fetus. An individual inheriting a single faulty tumor suppressor gene will not automatically develop cancer, but will have only one functional allele of that gene remaining in each cell of his or her body. If at any time during the life of such an indivdual, a mutation should occur in the remaining good allele of this gene *in any cell of the body*, a tumor will likely result.

So the development of a tumor requires the mutation of several genes. There must be at least one mutation in a gene activating cell division, an oncogene, that starts the cell down the pathway toward proliferation in the absence of an appropriate signal. But there must also be a mutation in one or more of the genes whose specific purpose is to detect and suppress such events: tumor-suppressor genes. The need to accumulate multiple mutations is one reason most cancers do not arise until relatively late in life.

The existence of oncogenes and tumor-suppressor genes was discovered through the study of cancer in animal models. In the past few years, single genes have been identified in humans which, when mutated, can cause a variety of cancers. Oncogene mutations are seen in a variety of different cancers; as expected, none of these cancers is of the hereditary type. Genes have also been identified in connection with cancers that have a strong hereditary basis: the BRCA-1 and BRCA-2 genes that cause certain breast and ovarian tumors, and the HNPCC-1 and -2 genes that cause colon cancers. All four of these genes are tumor suppressors. The BRCA genes are involved in a relatively small number of strongly hereditary breast cancers (five to ten percent of all breast cancers), and also predispose toward ovarian cancer. Defective alleles in either of these genes can result in a seventy-to ninety-percent incidence of cancer in affected individuals. (A recently discovered third gene, the AT gene, may also contribute significantly to strongly hereditary breast cancer.) The HNPCC genes, which are involved in DNA repair, are responsible for a highly hereditary form of colon cancer called *hereditary nonpolyposis colorectal cancer*, which accounts for about fifteen percent of all colorectal cancers in the United States. An estimated one million Americans are thought to carry the disease-causing alleles of these genes, and these individuals have a seventy-five-percent chance of developing colon cancer in their lifetimes. There is a second gene strongly predisposing to colorectal cancer, called the APC gene (for *adenomatous polyposis coli*).

The ability to screen for these genes in individuals with a strong family history of these cancers offers many advantages in terms of proactive treatments or lifestyle changes that can reduce the likelihood of disease; another advantage is early, intensive surveillance and prompt intervention once disease develops. However, this kind of *genetic screening* also creates a number of social and ethical problems, which we will explore in Chapter 13.

Sense and Antisense in Cancer

Molecular medicine provides a number of possibilities for treating cancers where a single gene—whether an oncogene or a tumor-suppressor gene—plays a dominant role. The most promising approach for cancers clearly involving a deranged oncogene is something referred to as the *antisense strategy*. The idea behind the antisense approach can be seen most clearly by recalling the structure of double-stranded DNA (see Figure 3-1). As we have seen, a gene is a defined linear sequence of nucleotides along one of the two DNA strands found at a given location on a chromosome. The nucleotide sequence defining the gene is referred to as the *sense* sequence for the gene. Notice that the nucleotide sequence along the opposing strand at the same location is clearly directed by the sequence defining the gene, but does not itself form a meaningful gene (i.e., it does not code for a protein.) But because its own sequence is the exact A-T, G-C complement of the gene itself, it is referred to as the *antisense* DNA sequence for this gene.

The messenger RNA produced when a given gene is transcribed is technically an antisense copy of the original gene, but because it is copied from the sense DNA strand it is, by convention, referred to as the *sense mRNA* for the gene. The stretch of DNA opposite a given gene (the antisense DNA) is not itself transcribed into RNA during transcription of the sense gene; its antisense composition would not encode appropriate promoter sequences needed to initiate transcription, and the protein sequence dictated would be nonsensical. But *if* the antisense DNA sequence *were* transcribed, the mRNA thus produced would be referred to as an *antisense mRNA*. This mRNA would not be translated, because it does not have sensible start codons, but it can be made in the laboratory.

The antisense strategy has been particularly successful with oncogene-induced tumors. A specially engineered antisense form of the errant oncogene is introduced into as many cancer cells as possible. The antisense gene contains promoter sequences allowing expression in the cancer cells being treated. When the transduced antisense gene and the endogenous sense gene produce their complementary sense and antisense mRNA molecules, these molecules will hybridize to produce a dsRNA molecule (Figure 9-1). This is at the heart of the antisense strategy. RNA molecules are not ordinarily found in the cell as double-stranded structures, and there are special enzymes in mammalian cells whose specific job it is to seek out and destroy any double-stranded RNA structures they en-counter.

This strategy is currently the subject of at least two clinical trials, and more are in the planning stages. The most common inappropriately activated oncogenes associated with human cancers belong to the so-called *ras oncogene* family. The proteins encoded by ras genes are usually found just under the cell's outer membrane, where they are involved in transmitting an external proliferative signal to the nucleus of the cell (Figure 9-2). An external signal (S) for cellular proliferation arrives at the cell and

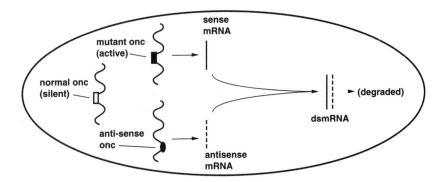

Figure 9-1. Antisense and cancer. The events shown here all take place in the nucleus of the cancer cell. The nucleus has one normal copy of the oncogene in question, and one mutant copy. The mutation causes the mutant oncogene to be transcribed when it should not be, driving the cell into unscheduled proliferation. An antisense copy of the gene is delivered to the nucleus of the cancer cell with an appropriate vector; the antisense oncogene is provided with a promoter that allows it to be continuously transcribed. The mRNA copies of the sense and antisense oncogenes are complementary to one another, and form a double-stranded RNA structure that is destroyed by enzymes in the cell.

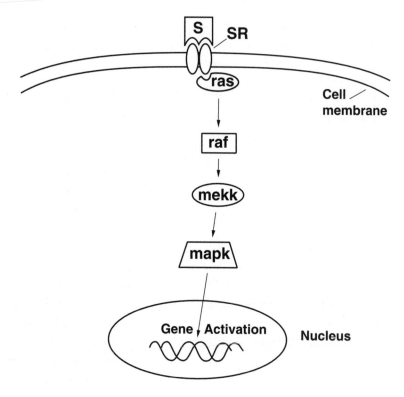

Figure 9-2. Oncogenes are signal transducers for cell proliferation.

binds to a signal receptor (SR) that is embedded in the cell membrane. The SR transmits this information to the inside of the cell. Ras is a molecule commonly found just below the membrane of many cells; it interacts with the SR if and only if the SR is engaged with S. (Different cells may have different SR that respond to different S, but all cells have a very limited number of internal signal transduction systems such as the ras pathway.) Ras activated by SR then starts a chain reaction of successive molecular changes involving other molecules like the ones shown in the Figure (raf, mekk, mapk); the last link in the chain is usually an intranuclear transcription factor that turns on genes involved in cell division. In many tumors, ras may be mutated into a form that acts on downstream components, such as raf, in the absence of an activating signal from SR occupied by S. In fact, any of the components of the pathway shown, beginning with SR and up through nuclear transcription factors, are potential oncogenes, in that a mutation in any one of them that leads to constant activation of the next molecule in the pathway could cause cancer. The aim of antisense treatment of such cells is to interfere with the production of the mutated, autoactivated ras, or any of the other oncogene products in the pathway.

Using a human lung-cancer cell-line with a prominent ras mutation (a single nucleotide alteration changing a single amino acid in the ras protein), one laboratory found that transduction of these cells with a ras antisense gene stopped cell division, both in vitro and in a nude mouse transplanted with the tumor. Based on strong preclinical laboratory evidence, a clinical trial has been approved for treating patients with advanced lung cancer. Patients who have had their tumors surgically reduced will have the remaining unresectable masses injected with a retroviral vector containing the ras antisense gene.

A second clinical trial is in progress using antisense treatment for another oncogene, called *fos*. This trial will focus on metastatic nonhereditary breast cancer, in which fos is often prominently expressed. The vector used in this trial is unique; it is itself a retrovirus that causes breast cancer in mice. The vector has been gutted to prevent its replication in human cells, but the endogenous promoter in this virus (which will be used to drive transcription of the antisense gene) can support the transcriptional machinery that is present in human breast cells, but not other cells. This means that even if the vector were somehow to get into other cells in the patient, it could not function, which provides an additional element of safety.

Rescuing Cancer from Itself: Gene Replacement Therapy for Cancer

One of the most intriguing possibilities offered by molecular medicine in the struggle against cancer is that in at least some cases, it may not be necessary to destroy the tumor at all. With our increased understanding of just how cell division is normally regulated in cells, it may be possible to rescue these otherwise healthy cells and redirect them to the useful functions nature intended. This represents a major change in mind-set about how cancer can be treated; it is representative perhaps of what can happen when a problem is understood rather than simply feared.

The same laboratory that initiated the ras-oncogene clinical trials has also generated a trial for the tumor suppressor gene *p53*. This gene is by far the most frequently mutated gene seen in human cancers; approximately half of all human tumors involve a mutated p53 gene. Altered p53 is particularly prevalent in lung, liver, and colon cancers, which in turn account for the majority of human cancers. The p53 gene is unusually interesting. In addition to its cancer associations, it is also involved in the body's response to radiation damage and viral infection. If a cell's DNA is damaged by radiation or chemical mutagens beyond the point where it can be repaired, p53 instructs the damaged cell to commit suicide. Many viruses that infect the body trigger cells to enter into abnormal cell division by neutralizing the cells' p53 supply. One of the functions of p53 is to guard against unwanted cell division; cells that enter into unscheduled cell division are also instructed by p53 to commit suicide. This is almost certainly the role of p53 that is defective in cancer, which would place p53 in the tumor-suppressor category of cancer-associated genes.

Because tumors caused by suppressor genes involve the loss of a critical gene product, the preferred molecular approach is standard gene therapy of the type used in CF or SCID: the replacement of a lost or mutated gene with a normal copy of that gene. In two human lung-cancer cell-lines with p53 mutations, transduction of the cells with a retroviral vector containing a normal p53 gene was again found to greatly suppress growth of the tumor cells. Interestingly, mixing a small proportion of p53-transduced cells with a larger number of untreated p53-deficient cancer cells led to growth suppression of the untransduced cells as well, suggesting some sort of "innocent-bystander" effect. The basis of this effect is not understood at present.

When human lung-cancer cells were injected into nude mice, sixty to eighty percent of the mice developed bronchial tumors. When the mice were injected at the same site with the p53-containing vector, up to 100 percent of the tumors (depending on the amount of p53 delivered) showed significant signs of tumor regression. Similar results were obtained using an adenovirus vector, which was also tested in combination with a standard chemotherapeutic agent for lung cancers called *cisplatin*. The combination of gene therapy and chemotherapy was extremely effective. The RAC and FDA have now approved protocols to test this procedure in human lung-cancer patients, and the first nine patients, all with advanced lung cancer, have been recruited into a clinical trial. The plan for Phase I studies is to inject the retroviral and adenoviral p53 vectors alone into these patients to study toxicity and efficiency of delivery. Initial results show that, one-to-three months after a single injection, no vector-related toxicity could be detected. Three patients have shown stabilization of their tumors, and three have shown significant tumor regression. In Phase II and III trials, which may involve patients with less advanced disease, the vectors will be combined with chemotherapy for further toxicity and efficacy studies.

The BRCA, HNPCC, and APC genes were discovered only recently, and their biology is not yet sufficiently understood to plan for clinical trials, but these may well come in the not-too-distant future. The problem will remain for antisense and gene replacement strategies that the majority of tumors involve more than one aberrant oncogene or tumor-suppresor gene. The vigorous cell division that sets in once a tumor begins to grow seems to facilitate the rapid accumulation of additional mutations in other genes that can contribute to cancer. Thus, although introduction of an oncogene antisense gene or a tumor-suppressor replacement gene may not be able to completely reverse any given tumor, the preclinical studies suggest that significant retardation of tumor growth may be achievable, particularly if the innocent-bystander phenomenon turns out to be more common than anyone dared to hope. And particularly if these treatments can be delivered when a cancer first arises, before multiple mutations have time to accumulate, treatment for a single mutation predominating early on may have a major effect. Standard gene therapy, for ras, p53, or other genes with prominent cancer associations may suppress tumor progression enough to tip the balance in favor of the body's immune system, or to allow other cancer therapies such as radiation and chemotherapy to become more effective.

Adoptive Immunotherapy

The second major approach using the techniques of molecular medicine to treat cancer is not aimed at the tumor per se, but rather at the immune system. There is abundant evidence from both human and animal studies over the past forty years that in many and perhaps most cases, the immune system does recognize tumor cells as abnormal and try to destroy them. In fact, it has been suggested that tumors may arise in our bodies fairly frequently; the ones that develop into clinically detectable cancers represent the relatively few that have managed to escape detection and destruction by the immune system. Attempts have been made in the past, using nongenetic means, to enhance the inherent immune responsiveness of human cancer patients to their tumors. Samples of tumor have been removed, dissociated into single cells, irradiated and reinjected at various sites in the body in an attempt to "immunize" patients against what is hopefully a more immunogenic (immune-response-inducing) form of their own tumor. Various substances thought to enhance immune responsiveness in general have been either injected directly into tumor masses, or mixed with the irradiated cells just prior to reinjection. Although never achieving long-term cures, enough of a response was seen in many cases to confirm the notion that the immune system, if somehow properly stimulated, could be a major factor in tumor defense.

A number of animal studies have also provided strong evidence that all of the various components of the immune system—antibodies, T cells, macrophages—are capable, working together under the right conditions, of clearing most kinds of tumor cells from the body most of the time. There are many ways in which tumors can evade immune destruction, but nearly all boil down to a failure to turn on immune defenses soon enough or strongly enough. It is very rare indeed for a tumor to escape by developing an inherent resistance to the immune mechanisms used to destroy aberrant cells. The development of a tumor in its earliest stages of growth involves a delicate balance between the tumor and the immune system; a slight tilt in one direction or the other may make the difference between an incident never perceived and a deadly tumor.

Recognition of the immune system's active role in combating tumors forms the basis for the second major molecular approach to managing cancer. This approach, called by a variety of names but perhaps most commonly *adoptive immunotherapy*, attempts to enhance the immune system's natural response to tumors mostly by manipulating the supply of cytokines called *interleukins*. As we know, interleukins are a collection of small protein molecules (e.g., IL-2) that control the activity of all the cells in the immune system. There are about two dozen interleukins, most of which are made by T cells, with a few also made by macrophages.

Animal studies have shown that interleukins administered *systemically* (e.g., by intravenous infusion) can exert powerful effects against a tumor's emergence, and that these effects are mediated through promoting vigorous and rapid immune responses. Unfortunately, the levels of these interleukins that were found to be required in animals such as mice and rats for an antitumor response would be too toxic in humans. When injected systemically at these levels, interleukins begin to affect the human immune system's normal function, and can interfere with other physiological compartments in the body such as the nervous system, bone marrow, or even the circulatory system. Nevertheless, there is good reason to think that, with appropriate modification, such an approach could work in humans. In some of the previous clinical studies, the higher doses of interleukins injected systemically have shown signs of stimulating an immune response against tumors. Moreover, when increased concentrations of the interleukins were introduced into the arterial circulation just upstream of the tumor itself (to achieve a higher local concentration at the site of the tumor without exposing the entire body to toxic levels of these agents), even more impressive effects were seen.

Studies such as these have led to the idea that if one could introduce interleukin genes into a tumor, and let the tumor cells themselves release these agents into the immediate vicinity, nearby immune cells such as T cells and macrophages might be stimulated to mount a more effective attack. Preliminary studies in animals have borne this out. A variety of different tumor types have been transduced with cytokines such as IL-2, IL-4, IL-7 and others that are known to stimulate various components of the immune system. The results have been impressive, leading in many cases to complete destruction of well-established and even metastatic tumors. Many of these studies have focussed on tumors that are highly resistant to standard cancer therapies such as radiation therapy or chemotherapy.

The RAC and FDA have now approved several clinical trials to explore this approach to treating cancer in humans. In fact the very next gene therapy trial carried out after Ashanti DeSilva's treatment for ADA-SCID was aimed at treating cancer using a retroviral vector containing a T cell cytokine called *tumor necrosis factor* (TNF). All of the trials approved so far are aimed at treating tumors that do not respond to conventional cancer therapy—metastatic malignant melanoma and some of the more refractory forms of lung cancer, for example. The most successful approach seems likely to be one in which some of the patient's cancer cells are removed, grown briefly in culture, and irradiated to stop growth (using radiation levels that would be lethal to normal cells in vivo). The irradiated cells are then transduced with a given cytokine gene and injected back into the patient, either at the site of the original tumor or elsewhere in the body. The irradiated cells cannot form a new tumor, but are able to express the cytokine transgene. The expectation is that through production of high local levels of the particular interleukin, these altered tumor cells will promote a vigorous immune response to the tumor. Once such a response has been generated, the immune elements involved, be they T cells, macrophages, or antibody, will be effective in the destruction of other tumor cells. Such an approach would thus be effective even against tumors that had already spread (*metastasized*) to other parts of the body.

The clinical trials currently underway are aimed at exploring the effectiveness of different cytokines against different tumors. The combinations under investigation are based on an analysis of the animal studies described above, and previous experience with introducing cytokines into cancer patients systemically. Typical of these trials is one currently underway at UCLA under the direction of Dr. James Economou. Preclinical studies in mice carried out by Economou and his colleague, Dr. William McBride, had shown that a line of highly tumorigenic fibrosarcoma cells transduced with a retroviral vector containing the gene for the T cell cytokine interleukin 7 (IL-7) were one-hundred to one-thousand-times less likely to develop into a tumor when implanted into mice than were unmodified cells. Moreover, mice that had been exposed to irradiated IL-7-transduced tumor cells were completely resistant to unmodified tumor cells. And injection of such cells into mice already carrying a tumor led to clearance of the tumor, including metastases to the lung. Subsequent analysis showed that mice that had been exposed to tumor cells producing and secreting IL-7 had developed a potent T-cell-based defense against the tumor. Additional studies showed that human tumor cells, including those from a malignant melanoma, could be transduced with this same vector, and that IL-7 gene expression was stable in such cells for many months.

On the basis of their extensive laboratory studies in animals and in human tumor cell lines, the UCLA group was granted permission to carry out a Phase I study to test the value of treating human melanoma patients with their own IL-7-modified tumor cells. In this particular study, instead of transducing each patient's own tumor cells with a retrovirus carrying the IL-7 gene, the researchers have prepared a standardized melanoma tumor cell line (M24) that is stably transfected with the IL-7 gene, and reliably secretes ample amounts of IL-7. A sample of the patient's tumor is removed, dissociated into single cells, and mixed with M24 cells in various ratios. The cell mixture is then irradiated and reinjected into the patient at a subcutaneous site on the abdomen. The IL-7 released at the site by the M24 cells should stimulate an immune response to both the M24 melanoma cells and the patient's own tumor. The immune defenses thus mobilized can then circulate throughout the body and attack melanoma cells wherever they are found. In future trials, the investigators will likely also include the patient's own IL-7-transduced tumor cells as part of the immunizing mixture.

Future trials, using IL-7 and other candidate cytokines, will examine questions relating to methods of administration, or the timing of treatment. Patients in Phase I trials all have advanced disease that has proved unresponsive to standard medical therapies. Phase II and III trials will involve patients with earlier stage disease, where gene therapy can be integrated with other treatments, rather than using gene therapy only after all other treatments have failed. For example, experiments in laboratory animals suggest that when the tumor burden is reduced as a result of initial surgical, radiation or chemotherapy treatment, the immune system may be naturally in a state of "rebound," and better able to respond once again to the tumor challenge. Obviously when tumors recur after treatment, the balance has tipped once again in favor of the tumor and against the immune system. But this interim period, between treatment-induced tumor regression and re-emergence of the tumor, would seem to be an ideal time to introduce immune-system-enhancing elements into the tumor through gene therapy. This approach to treatment should begin taking place once the current round of Phase I trials are completed.

When All Else Fails . . .

For those tumors not treatable by gene transfer or by immune stimulation, molecular medicine offers one other option: the embedding of genes in tumor cells that make them more sensitive to treatment with anticancer drugs. One of the more intriguing variants of this approach involves one of the most deadly and untreatable of all human cancers: brain tumors. Over 30,000 people die each year in the U.S. from various brain cancers. It is the third-leading cancer cause of death among people in their prime of life, fifteen to thirty-four years of age. The brain is a histologically complex organ, and there are many different types of brain tumors. Among the most deadly is one called *glioblastoma multiforme* (GBM). When all three weapons in the oncologists' standard repertoire—surgery, radiation, and chemotherapy—are brought to bear against GBM, survival is still a matter of weeks or months at best. If ever there was a disease in desperate need of a new approach to treatment, it is GBM: mortality from this form of cancer is essentially one hundred percent.

A scheme originally proposed by Dr. Ken Culver and Dr. Michael Blaese at NIH takes advantage of the experience gained in previous gene therapy trials for SCID and CF, and adds some completely new and highly imaginative twists. The overall strategy is to introduce a gene called *Hstk* into tumor cells, and then to treat the patient with a drug called *gancyclovir*. Rapidly dividing cells that express the Hstk gene are extraordinarily sensitive to gancyclovir; if exposed to it, they will die.

The Hstk gene itself is not a human gene; it comes from a common virus infecting humans called *Herpes simplex*. Type I herpes causes the "cold sores" that periodically break out on lips, nostrils and the surrounding skin. Type II herpes, also known as "genital herpes," causes blister-like sores in the genital region. The tk gene carried by these herpes viruses encodes an enzyme called *thymidine kinase*, which chemically alters nucleotides in a way that makes them more useful for synthesis of viral DNA. However, thymidine kinase also chemically alters the drug gancyclovir (itself a nucleotide analog) in a way that makes it a poison for rapidly dividing mammalian cells. That is why gancyclovir (and its chemical analog *acyclovir*) are effective against tk-bearing viruses such as Herpes.

The idea of using Hstk in gene therapy arose when the NIH group was considering the use of retroviral vectors in connection with the first ADA-SCID trials. Everyone using retroviruses to treat human beings is haunted by the possibility that a retroviral vector might cause an insertional mutation in one of the oncogenes or tumor-suppressor genes, thus leading to the formation of a tumor. The chances are very slim, but nevertheless real. Culver and Blaese came up with the idea of including Hstk in their overall vector design so that if one of the transduced cells did become cancerous, they would be able to eradicate the resulting tumor with gancyclovir. In effect, any cell developing into a tumor would commit suicide.

It was only a small jump to realize that what they were proposing as a safeguard for ADA-SCID gene therapy could have tremendous value for treating cancer in general. Thus they set out to explore the possibility of inserting a "suicide gene" (Hstk) into a disabled MoMLV retroviral vector, similar to the one used for delivery of the ADA gene, for general use in cancer treatment. Since retroviruses infect only dividing cells to begin with, tumor cells should be selectively targeted in a region of the body where tumor is growing; very little of the vector DNA should get into surrounding nondividing cells. Moreover, gancyclovir itself, when "activated" by the tk gene product, is only toxic to dividing cells.

But how does one deliver the viral vector and its passenger suicide gene to a brain tumor in the first place? An ex vivo approach is obviously not practical, and the target in this case is not part of an epithelial surface with connections to airways, lungs, and so forth. Viruses cannot be delivered through the blood because they would have no way of knowing, as they cruise inside blood vessels, just where in the body they are; even if they did know, they would have no way of getting out of the bloodstream. Furthermore, even if one could find a way to deliver viral vectors to the tumor, how could they be delivered to every single cell within a tumor mass? We know only too well from experience with other modes of cancer treatment that if even one tumor cell is left behind, it will surely give rise in time to a new and possibly more deadly tumor.

The solution to these problems proposed by Culver and his colleagues is truly ingenious. They decided not to inject the viral vector itself into the tumor mass, but rather, infect packaging cells that *produce* the vector (Figure 9-3a). Packaging cells are equipped with copies of the genes removed from the viral vector to prevent replication. When transduced with a replication-deficient retroviral genome containing a passenger gene, packaging cells are able to convert it into an intact, infectious retrovirus and release it into the surrounding medium. Moreover, the packaging cells can go on releasing retroviruses for long periods of time. The retroviruses produced by the packaging cells are able to infect surrounding cells, if they are dividing; once inside these cells, the retroviral provirus is able to transcribe the passenger gene, but is unable to reproduce itself. So the basic idea behind the Culver and Blaese approach is to implant tiny gene factories—packaging cells—in the middle of the tumor, and let them pump a steady stream of retroviruses carrying suicide genes that can infect the surrounding tumor mass. In effect, tumor cells are being asked to take up the vector and produce their own anti-tumor chemotherapeutic drugs. Both the delivery vector (a retrovirus) and the

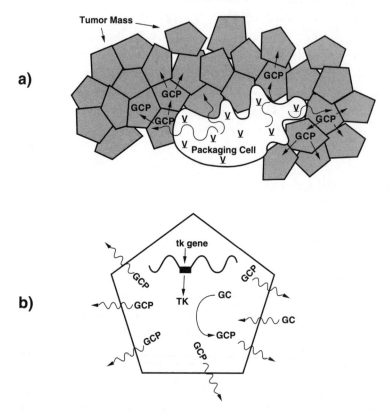

Figure 9-3. Packaging cells and the "innocent bystander effect." Packaging cells producing the recombinant retrovirus containing a tk gene are injected into the middle of a tumor mass (a). Infectious viral particles (v) are released into some of the surrounding cells. Since the virus cannot replicate outside the packaging cell, it does not spread very far into the tumor. Gancyclovir (GC) has been administered to the patient intravenously, and reaches the cells within the tumor. Inside those tumor cells transduced by the viral vector (b), the tk gene product (TK) converts gancyclovir into a phosphorylated form (GCP) that shuts down DNA synthesis in any dividing cell, causing that cell to die. GCP is able to pass from one cell to another throughout the tumor, eventually reaching all the tumor cells, thus greatly amplifying the effect of the relatively few cells transduced by the viral vector.

suicide gene (Hstk) are selected to act only on rapidly dividing cells; in the brain, this could only be tumor cells.

The pre-clinical studies in animals using this approach were extremely promising. A tumor similar to GBM was deliberately implanted into the brain of laboratory rats. After five days of growth, the tumor masses of some rats were carefully injected with a minute quantity of packaging cells containing a retroviral genome with an embedded Hstk gene. Five days later the rats began receiving twice-daily intravenous injections of gancyclovir. All of the rats that were not treated in this fashion died of their tumors within four weeks. Every single rat receiving an injection of packaging cells, followed by gancyclovir injections, showed startling and rapid regression of their tumors; eighty percent recovered completely. When the rats recovering from their tumors were later sacrificed and their brains examined microscopically, there was no sign of tumor cells anywhere in the brain. Nor was there any sign of damage to healthy brain cells in the region of the former tumor.

It turns out that this technique worked much better than the investigators could have imagined. A close analysis of the cancerous rat brains during the process of clearing the tumor showed that in fact not all of the tumor cells had taken up the retrovirus with its tk gene. Even when only five percent or so of the tumor cells were invaded by the vector, all of the tumor cells died. This is precisely what is needed (but what almost no one dared to hope for) in the treatment of cancer by gene therapy: complete elimination of a tumor with less-than-total transduction of the cells. But what was the basis of this innocent-bystander killing of uninfected tumor cells? There appear to be at least two explanations, neither anticipated — but both certainly welcomed — by the Culver-Blaese research team. It seems that before the tumor cells died from the combination of Hstk and gancyclovir, they managed to pass some of their "activated" gancyclovir to surrounding cells (Figure 9-3b). Exactly how this happens is not entirely clear, but it has the happy result that one tumor cell infected with the delivery vector can actually end up killing not only itself, but a number of surrounding tumor cells as well.

A second possible source of the innocent-bystander effect involves the blood vessels serving the tumor. Tumors such as GBM grow extremely rapidly, and to sustain their extraordinary growth rate they must be provided with blood and its precious nutrients and oxygen. Such tumors release chemical signals that recruit nearby blood vessels, causing them to enlarge and expand by rapid cell division to keep up with the tumors' needs; thus in many instances the cells forming the blood vessels are dividing almost as rapidly as the tumor itself. This in turn makes the cells of the blood vessels as susceptible to retroviral infection and the destructive action of gancyclovir as the tumor cells. When the rats' brains were examined in the midst of the tumor-destruction process, one of the most prominent features was numerous ruptured blood vessels scattered throughout the tumor. The resulting deprivation of food and oxygen would be absolutely lethal for a rapidly growing tumor.

Culver and Blaese teamed up with Dr. Edward Oldfield, the chief of neurosurgery at the National Cancer Institute, to treat human patients with GBM. Theirs would be the first proposal for the direct introduction of retroviral vectors into human beings in vivo, rather than ex vivo. But based on the extraordinary findings in the animal studies, and given the exceedingly poor prognosis of GBM in humans, the RAC and FDA approved a Phase I trial for the Hstk-gancyclovir strategy in August 1992. The first patients, all with advanced disease that had failed standard treatment, were recruited into clinical trials almost immediately. The tumors were located using sophisticated magnetic resonance imaging (MRI) techniques. With the patient under total anesthesia, the MRI images were used to guide a thin needle through a hole in the skull and into the tumor mass. Varying numbers of infected packaging cells were introduced through the needle in single or multisite injections. The patients were observed closely for forty-eight hours post-surgery, and again as the gancyclovir treatments began. (Experiments in animals with advanced tumors of various kinds have shown that if the tumor is first reduced surgically, treatment with a suicide vector is much more effective in clearing up residual tumor.)

As of mid-1996, fifteen patients have been entered into this study. Although the results have not yet appeared in the medical literature, a few preliminary findings have surfaced informally at scientific meetings. The procedure has caused no serious toxicity or undesirable side effects in any of the patients treated. Approximately twenty-five percent of the patients have shown measurable tumor reduction, even though this is only a Phase I trial. Several are alive well beyond the period of time normally expected for patients with their disease. In some patients, changes in the tumor cells resulting from previous radiation treatments appeared to block the efficacy of gene therapy, and not all of the injections reached their targets. But this is only a Phase I trial, intended to gather precisely this type of information. Future Phase II and III trials will hopefully include patients with earlier stage disease, with the gene therapy taking place earlier in the overall course of treatment.

The RAC and FDA have been sufficiently impressed with formal progress reports from the NIH team to allow three additional medical centers to begin their own Phase I trials. Culver has begun another program at the University of Iowa, where he moved in 1993. At least one European center has initiated an identical trial. The idea of using packaging cells has now been extended to other brain tumors, and is being actively explored for delivering suicide genes to other solid tumors as well. Variants of the basic protocol, using adenovirus rather than a retrovirus as the delivery vector, are being explored. Since the Hstk strategy is only effective in rapidly dividing cells anyway, the use of retrovirus as a delivery vector offers no particular advantage. And, in the case of cancer treatment, the tendency of adenovirus to induce an inflammatory reaction against transduced cells is actually a plus rather than a negative. Preclinical studies in live animals with human tumor cells are in an advanced stage for ovarian and nonhereditary colon cancers, and for malignant melanoma. It seems very likely that protocols for treating these diseases in humans will be submitted in the next two years.

Playing the Endgame

Billions of years ago, when the earliest living cells made the transition from a prokaryotic to a eukaryotic state, one of the most important changes wrought was in the state of their chromosomes. Prokaryotic cells such as bacteria have a single copy of a single chromosome, which is kept in a closed circular form. The more evolutionarily advanced eukaryotic cells, which eventually gave rise to complex multicellular animals such as humans, opened these circular structures into linear chromosomes of the type we have today. Opening up the chromosomes created a small problem, however: the tendency of the linear chromosomes' sticky ends to cause random end-to-end chromosomal clumping, making chromosomal replication and cell division extremely difficult. Cells solved this problem by creating special "capping" structures at the end of each linearized chromosome called *telomeres*. Telomeres are themselves DNA, but of a special composition and "shape" that inhibits rather than promotes chromosomal clumping.

One of the interesting things about telomeric DNA is that it is not replicated with the rest of the chromosomal DNA during cell division. In those cells that must undergo many cell divisions as a normal part of their life history, telomeric DNA is added to the ends of chromosomes after each division by a special enzyme called telomerase. But this enzyme is virtually undetectable in most normal adult human somatic cells. Thus one of the current theories of aging is that we gradually lose telomeric DNA at the ends of our chromosomes until they clump together and are no longer able to divide. Cell machinery put into place to detect DNA abnormalities then shuts the cell down, greatly accelerating the aging process. Indeed, in most eukaryotic cells, including humans, telomeres do get shorter with increasing age. But the rather startling observation was made that in cancer cells taken from an older person, in whom telomerase activity was undetectable, the telomerase activity had shot up to levels ordinarily seen only in a very young person. It is now thought that the reversal of declining telomerase activity is one of the genetic "tricks" played by cancer cells to escape the senescence that ordinarily seals the fate of any eukaryotic cell over time; it is part of the secret of immortality discovered by cancer cells.

Once this was realized, researchers began to search for a way to interfere with the enhanced telomerase activity in cancer cells. They discovered a potential weak spot in the way telomerase works to add the capping structures to chromosomes (Figure 9-4.) Like all enzymes, telomerase is a protein. But telomerase is very unusual in that it has appended to it a stretch of RNA that serves as a "template" for the creation of a DNA-based telomeric structure. Telomeres in humans consist of multiple repeats of the DNA motif GGGTTA. Human telomerase contains an RNA stretch that partially overlaps with this sequence, and contains information for its extension. What researchers have found is that by flooding the nucleus with free copies of the telomere motif, telomerase becomes so engaged with the free DNA pieces that it cannot carry out its normal task of extending the real telomeres. The challenge is now to figure out a way to deliver excess amounts of "minimotifs" to cancer cells in vivo. One way might be to deliver a gene encoding multiple copies of this

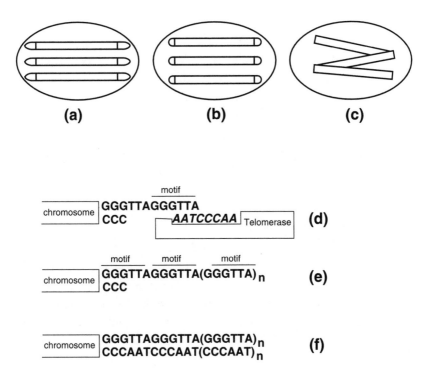

Figure 9-4. Telomeres and cancer. Telomeres, which cap each end of each chromosome, become shorter with age (a, b), possibly causing chromosomes to clump together (c). Cancer cells, on the other hand, revert to a "younger" stage of the cell (a). Telomeres are added to the end of each chromosome at the end of each cell division by a special enzyme called telomerase (d). The end of each chromosome has one copy of the telomere motif; telomerase has a short segment of DNA attached to it that is the antisense of this motif. The enzyme attaches to the end of the chromosome, and a special form of DNA polymerase fills in the strand with the motif DNA. This process is repeated over and over resulting in multiple repeats of the motif (e). Another form of DNA polymerase then fills in the opposite strand to complete the telomere structure (f).

motif in the same way that antisense genes are delivered. Although far from being ready for the clinic, some very interesting preclinical trials in mice with cancer are currently underway, and the results are highly encouraging.

The foregoing are but a few of the imaginative approaches being explored by "molecular oncologists" to apply the techniques of molecular biology to cancer treatment. Other approaches are being explored as well. One interesting variation is the genetic modification not of the tumor cells themselves, but of bone-marrow cells. Bone marrow is extremely sensitive to some of the drugs used in cancer chemotherapy. Many of these drugs selectively target rapidly dividing cells, because tumors are composed of just such cells; unfortunately, so is bone marrow (except for the stem cells). Oncologists are often prevented from using levels of these drugs that would eradicate the tumor because of bone-marrow damage. One way around this would be to transduce bone marrow cells with genes that confer resistance — rather than sensitivity — to these chemotherapeutic drugs, thus allowing the physician to administer the higher levels needed.

Yet another possible genetic manipulation that might affect tumor growth would be to take advantage of the fact tumor cells need huge numbers of blood vessels to bring in food and oxygen. Tumor cells secrete two types of factors, those that stimulate vascularization (*angiogenesis*) annd those that inhibit this process. The overall blood supply to the tumor will depend on the balance between these factors. Some of the anti-angiogenic factors are proteins. It may well be possible to remove a few tumor cells, transduce them with a gene encoding an anti-angiogenic protein, and then reintroduce the altered cells into the tumor mass (after irradiation, of course). The protein factor would be released into the surrounding tumor, cutting off the blood supply, and affected portions of the tumor would quickly die from starvation.

Cancer treatment in the twenty-first century will be very different from what it is today. No one is ready yet to discontinue any of the present treatment strategies. But those treatments were devised at a time when we simply did not understand what cancer is. Our new view of cancer has also led to a change in how we think cancer might be most effectively treated. Cancer cells are no longer viewed as mysterious, incomprehensible rogue cells that must be bludgeoned to death. They are seen as generally healthy cells that have simply developed a problem with controlling cell division. Now that we understand a great deal more about how cell division works than we did twenty years ago, we understand a great deal more about cancer itself. That doesn't make cancer any less dangerous as a disease, but it does provide an opportunity to rethink the way in which we try to treat it, particularly in combination with the new tools of molecular medicine.

Using molecular medicine to treat cancer is different from using standard gene therapy to correct hereditary monogenic diseases, because cancer is normally more complex than a single gene defect. And in treating cancer it is critical that ultimately every single cancer cell be either brought under control or destroyed. Any remaining cell can give rise to a new and even more resistant tumor. Thus for cancer, it is unlikely that gene therapy will displace other current cancer treatment modalities completely, where such modalities exist, but will rather serve as an additional and in many cases very effective adjunct form of treatment. For most cancers, several forms of treatment are normally used to achieve this goal: surgery, where possible, often followed by radiation therapy and/or chemotherapy, the latter frequently involving several different drugs. The present inefficiency of therapeutic gene delivery makes it unlikely that gene therapy would ever be able to eliminate every cancer cell on its own, although the "packaging-cell strategy" suggests that in certain situations gene therapy may go quite far in that direction. But most importantly, it must be remembered that many cancers respond poorly or not at all to current standard cancer therapies: malignant melanoma, and certain brain and kidney tumors, for example. These have in fact been precisely the cancers treated so far with the experimental methods we have looked at here; for these cancers, gene therapy may offer new hope to patients who would otherwise have a very poor outlook.

The very complexities of cancer, such as its multigenic nature, can be an advantage for molecular medicine; there are just that many more ways to attack the problem. The numerous clinical trials currently underway based on molecular-genetic techniques reflects this plethora of opportunities (Table 9-1). As molecular biologists continue to focus their attention on this multifaceted disease, we are likely to see even more imaginative approaches to its treatment and, in many cases, eradication in the near future.

Table 9-1. *Molecular medicine and cancer.*

(The clinical trials listed below represent a partial list of those already in progress. Numbers in parentheses are the number of currently approved trials for that cancer; some institutions are running multiple trials on the same cancer)

Cancer:	Participating Institutions:
Malignant Melanoma (6)	UCLA; Duke University; University of Michigan; NIH; University of Pittsburgh; Sloan Kettering

Table 9-1. *(continued)*

Cancer:	Participating Institutions:
Prostate (5)	Sloan-Kettering; University of Tennessee; National Naval Medical Center; Duke University; Baylor College of Medicine
Leukemia (2)	University of Minnesota; Northwestern University; St. Jude's Children's Hospital; M.D. Anderson Hospital; Indianna
UniversityOvarian (5)	NIH; University of Alabama; Vanderbilt University
Colon (3)	Georgetown University; Cornell Medical Center; Medical University of South Carolina
Myeloma	University of Arkansas; NIH
Renal Carcinoma	UCLA; Sloan-Kettering
Hodgkin's Lymphoma	St. Jude's Children's Hospital
Neuroblastoma (3)	St. Jude's Children's Hospital
Breast (2)	M.D. Anderson Hospital; NIH
Glioma	UCLA
Head and Neck Carcinoma (2)	University of Cinncinatti; Johns Hopkins University
Bladder	University of California (San Francisco)
Brain	NIH

10

Molecular Medicine and AIDS

AIDS (aquired immune deficiency syndrome) is probably more indelibly impressed on contemporary consciousness than any disease in modern history. It is truly the equivalent of the Black Death of the Middle Ages, or of smallpox just a few generations ago. One million Americans — and twenty million human beings worldwide — are estimated to be infected with the causative pathogen of AIDS — the human immunodeficiency virus (HIV). Fifteen percent of those infected are women. A quarter of a million Americans have already died of AIDS; without a major breakthrough in treatment, all but a tiny handful of those currently infected will die. They will die for one simple reason: HIV will have destroyed their T cells.

The consequences of destruction of the T cell arm of the immune response became clear in our earlier discussions of SCID. In higher mammals such as humans, T cells have come to play an increasingly dominant role in immune defenses; diseases that cripple T cells have unusually widespread effects. The various forms of SCID affect only children; AIDS affects mostly adults, but can also affect children if they somehow become exposed to HIV. The results are the same in either case: loss of immune function, and infection with opportunistic pathogens, followed by certain death if the disease is untreated. In the case of SCID, a small number of children have been saved in the past by bone-marrow transplants. Bone marrow transplants are useless in AIDS because the new-bone marrow cells coming into the body would be reinfected by residual HIV. For SCID patients, molecular medicine may provide a much needed adjunct to standard therapies such as bone-marrow transplantation; for AIDS patients, gene therapy may just possibly be the only hope.

HIV is a retrovirus; like all viruses, it is nothing more than a string of nucleic acids wrapped up in a few proteins. It is unable to reproduce itself on its own; to do so it must infect a living cell, and exploit that cell's materials and energy to make more of the virus. Viruses are unusually adept at binding to and entering cells. They do this through macromolecules on their surface that recognize and attach to complementary macromolecules on the surface of living cells. One of the proteins making up the coat of HIV is a glycoprotein (a protein that contains sugar molecules) called *gp120*. HIV uses the gp120 protein to bind to the cell it is going to infect. The gp120 protein specifically recognizes and binds to CD4, which is found on the surface of helper T cells. As the name suggests, helper T cells are very important in promoting the reactivity of other cells of the immune system, and they do this through the production of chemical messages called interleukins. It is the predilection of HIV to bind to CD4 molecules on helper T cells that ultimately makes this virus so deadly. The ability to bind to T cells is not a general property of retroviruses; other retroviruses have surface receptors that target them to a variety of different cells.

HIV behaves exactly as the retroviruses we have seen previously. It binds to a cell, sheds its protein coat, and inserts its single strand of RNA into the cell. This ss-RNA is converted by the enzyme reverse transcriptase into ds-DNA, which then integrates into the host genome as a provirus. (HIV carries multiple copies of the reverse transcriptase enzyme inside its coat for use once it successfully penetrates a cell.) And therein lies one of the fundamental similarities, yet one of the fundamental differences, between the role of retroviruses in the treatment of SCID and their role in AIDS pathology: the genes that make up the normal HIV genome *cause* the disease. These genes become embedded in the DNA of infected cells, and they are there permanently (or at least until the cell dies of infection, after releasing hundreds of new viruses). No treatment for AIDS can ever remove the HIV genes from an infected cell; the challenge for molecular oncologists is somehow to neutralize their effect. In gene therapy for SCID, we use a disabled retrovirus to deliver "good" genes for exactly the reason that makes HIV so deadly: permanent insertion of retroviral DNA (plus any passenger genes) into the host genome. But in that case we want to promote and protect, as long as possible, the continued function of the retroviral DNA containing the passenger gene.

One of the peculiarities of HIV is that after it infects a cell, an unusually large number of mistakes are made during reverse transcription, in the form of incorporation of incorrect nucleotides into DNA. This results in an unusually high mutation rate of the resulting proviral DNA and changes in many of the HIV proteins. Most of these mutations are likely to be deleterious to the virus, but that does not matter. The virus reproduces so rapidly inside a living cell that errors are affordable, as long as a few functional viruses are made in the process. The advantage to HIV of this "hypermutation" is that on occasion these mutations will lead a cell to produce slightly altered forms of the virus that are even more effective in replicating or spreading throughout the body than the virus originally infecting the cell. Mutations in the coat proteins of the virus are also important in helping HIV escape destruction by the immune system. As rapidly as the immune system can learn to recognize and attack one form of the virus, other forms emerge. Eventually one arises that simply overwhelms the body's defenses, and full-blown AIDS is the result.

Why does infection with HIV, alone among all viral infections, result in an acquired immune deficiency? In terms of the human immune system, the single most important fact about HIV is its ability to infect selectively and ultimately to destroy human helper T cells. HIV is also more effective at infecting cells in that, unlike most retroviruses, HIV can infect cells that are not actively dividing. From a clinical point of view, it has been clear from the start that one of the most reliable predictors for the progression of AIDS as a disease is the level of viable CD4 T cells remaining in the blood. CD4 T cells affect virtually every phase of our immune responsiveness. In one's wildest imagination, one could not possibly pick a worse cell to serve as the target for an infectious virus.

To this day no one knows exactly how HIV kills CD4 T cells. We do know that many strains of HIV can kill CD4 T cells directly, (i.e., they are *cytotoxic*). CD4 T cells incubated in a test tube with such HIV strains will die, in the absence of any other agent. Inside the body, HIV probably does kill at least some CD4 T cells directly. But some of the deadliest HIV strains are not cytotoxic to T cells. How, then, do such strains lead to a loss of CD4 T cells? One possibility is that HIV may also induce in its victims a form of immunological fratricide. Remember that a major task of the immune system is to rid the body of virally infected cells. If the infected cells are themselves part of the immune system, the same rules apply. T cell-mediated killing of HIV-infected cells in the brain is very likely responsible for the neurological deficits seen in many AIDS patients. So why wouldn't T cells do the same to each other? They do. CD8 T cells that kill CD4 T cells infected with HIV have in fact been demonstrated during AIDS progression. As in so many other situations of immunopathology, we realize that the immune system is simply following a predetermined program. T cells continue to lash out according to instructions, felling anything and everything in their path that is perceived to be compromised—even themselves.

The only AIDS treatment currently approved for standard use is aimed at preventing HIV from expressing itself in cells, and centers around a single type of drug, the best known example of which is azidothymidine (AZT), also known by its trade name, Zidovudine. Although there are now more than a dozen drugs approved by the Food and Drug Administration for treating various aspects of HIV infection, AZT and related compounds are the only ones that have made a significant impact on patient survival. AZT was originally developed as a potential anticancer drug, but was approved for treating AIDS patients in 1987. Since its introduction, AZT treatment has effectively doubled the lifespan of persons diagnosed with AIDS—unfortunately, only from about one year to two. But that is a start.

AZT is a slightly altered form of the nucleic acid, thymidine. When AZT is incorporated into DNA in place of thymidine, all further DNA synthesis stops. The advantage of AZT is that normal cells in the body cannot use AZT very well in place of thymidine. But viruses such as HIV <u>can</u> use AZT. If AZT is present in a cell when HIV is trying to make DNA copies of its RNA genetic blueprint, AZT will be preferentially incorporated into the copies, and viral DNA synthesis is quickly halted. However, AZT has no effect on expression of proviral HIV DNA already incorporated into the host-cell genome. Moreover, because of its incredibly fast mutation rate, HIV will eventually evolve strains able to use AZT *without* inhibiting DNA synthesis. Tests have shown that HIV strains present in the same patient after a year of treatment with AZT are over one hundred times more resistant to AZT than were the strains present before treatment was started. Further drug treatment at that point is completely useless. So AZT simply buys a little time; the eventual outcome is unchanged.

The AZT-related drugs currently in use include ddI (*dideoxyinosine*) and ddC (*dideoxycytosine*); both act in much the same way as AZT, but have fewer side effects. AZT can cause headaches, nausea, and a severe form of anemia, all of which limit the doses that can be used. Only about half of all AIDS patients can tolerate AZT for more than a year. The drugs ddI and ddC are less toxic, but they, too, drive HIV to mutate into drug-resistant forms. The current strategy is to give combinations of AZT and ddI or ddC, in the hope that it will be much harder for HIV to develop two simultaneous drug-resistant mutations. This may buy additional time, but again the eventual outcome will not likely change. Drug treatment at present for AIDS is thus purely *palliative* (granting temporary relief from symptoms), and not at all curative.

A highly promising drug still in the experimental stages, but ready for general release in the very near future, is something called *protease inhibitor*. When the HIV provirus begins to produce viral proteins in an infected cell, all of the proteins are initially strung together end to end, and must be cleaved apart in order to produce the individual proteins needed to make new viruses. This is the job of a special enzyme called a *protease*. Several drug companies have now come up with potent inhibitors of this enzyme, and the initial results are highly promising, especially when the inhibitors are used in combination with AZT or its derivatives (in so-called "drug cocktails"). It would be considerably more difficult for HIV strains to evolve that are resistant to both types of drug, since their mode of action is completely different. However, given the rapid rate of mutation of HIV, double mutants are not at all inconceivable (in fact they have already been seen in the laboratory), and such doubly-resistant strains will be particularly deadly, because by definition they are already resistant to the most powerful drugs at our disposal.

Given the nearly one-hundred-percent lethality of AIDS, and the lack of truly effective therapeutic approaches for controlling HIV expression and function, aggressive development of novel treatment strategies is still desperately needed. Approaches based on molecular medicine are under active investigation in laboratories all over the world. The underlying rationale for these approaches is that this disease is caused by genes that, through retroviral integration into the human genome, have become the equivalent of endogenous human disease-causing genes, and the affected cells can be treated accordingly. Like most cancers, AIDS is not a disease caused by a single defective gene that can be replaced with a good copy of a known human gene. Thus straightforward gene replacement approaches used for treating diseases such as SCID and CF may not be useful in treating AIDS. But as with cancer, the very complexities of HIV reproduction and of its interaction with CD4 cells may be its Achilles' heel. Every step in the generation of HIV offers a potential target for interference using the techniques of molecular medicine. In principle, it should be easier to treat AIDS than cancer using these techniques. HIV infects only bone-marrow-derived cells, so therapeutic genes can be delivered ex vivo, as with SCID. Moreover, since transduced cells will clearly have a survival advantage in treated patients, it will not be necessary to transduce every cell involved in the disease.

Gene-based strategies for treating AIDS fall into several distinct categories. Each category is based on the idea that we may never be able completely to rid HIV-infected patients of their virus. Rather, we must focus on neutralizing the virus's ability to replicate or to express itself in an infected cell. Some of the many approaches currently being explored for AIDS treatment are described in the following sections.

AIDS and Antisense

The antisense strategy for managing oncological disease is also one of the molecular approaches proposed for treating AIDS. The idea behind the anti-sense approach to treating HIV infection is to select an HIV gene critical to the function of this virus within an infected cell, and to introduce into infected cells (either before or after infection) an antisense DNA copy of that gene. This specially constructed "mirror-image gene" will include the requisite upstream promoter sequences allowing recognition and transcription by the host cell. The sense gene of the virus and the transduced antisense gene will produce their respective sense and antisense mRNAs. These will hybridize together to produce dsRNA molecules, which will be destroyed by the cell.

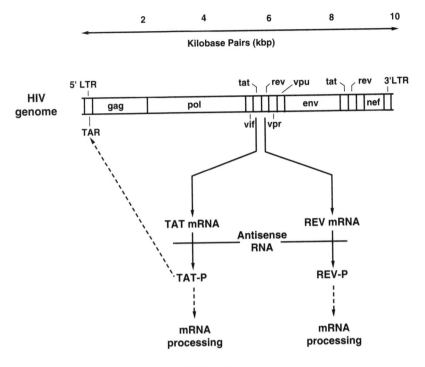

Figure 10-1. Antisense inhibition of HIV replication.

An example of how this has worked in HIV-infected cells in the laboratory is shown in Figure 10-1. The HIV genes Rev and Tat encode proteins that are critical in the early stages of HIV infection; without these proteins, the rest of the viral genes cannot be read. The Tat gene is first copied into Tat mRNA, and the Tat mRNA is then "translated" into the Tat protein. The Tat protein searches out and binds to a recognition element called TAR placed in front of each HIV gene, which allows them to be read and their protein products used to produce new viruses. Rev is equally important. It encodes a protein that helps transport the instructions for HIV proteins (the ones induced by Tat) out of the nucleus where they can be translated into HIV proteins. Without Rev, these instructions simply pile up unread in the nucleus and are eventually destroyed.

Antisense copies of the Rev gene have been transduced into human CD4 T cells grown in the laboratory, using replication-deficient retroviral vectors. The Rev antisense gene was expressed, and produced an antisense Rev mRNA, which promptly began "mopping up" Rev sense mRNA molecules within the nucleus. Thus Rev mRNA could not be translated into Rev protein, which greatly impaired processing and transport of the other HIV mRNAs. The cells quickly stopped producing infectious HIV particles. The cells were still there, and they were still HIV-infected, but they were simply unable to produce the proteins necessary to assemble new virus.

Similar results have been obtained with Tat. Antisense Tat mRNA vectors have been produced that greatly reduce the translation of the Tat protein in infected cells. Because the Tat protein is critical for inducing transcription of all the other HIV genes, the production of HIV proteins (including Rev) was correspondingly diminished. Even more effective have been antisense vectors for the Tat-binding TAR regions themselves. TAR is a promoter region, and is not normally transcribed into an RNA molecule. However, vectors can be made that contain a TAR sense DNA sequence, with a normal cellular promoter that will be recognized by the cell's own transcription machinery. The resulting TAR sense RNA can bind directly to the TAR region itself, blocking access by the Tat protein.

Clinical trials to explore the efficacy of TAR antisense treatment are currently underway at the NIH. Trials using antisense Tat and Rev will likely get under way in the near future at other centers. Before examining how the NIH trial is designed, however, we must look at a second molecular strategy for dealing with HIV infection, because the NIH study incorporates both in the same delivery vector.

The "Dominant-Negative" Strategy

A second approach to interfering with HIV reproduction in infected cells is based on something called the *dominant-negative* effect. This term describes a type of mutation frequently seen in normal cells (Figure 10-2). When one of the two alleles of a given gene is mutated, a slightly altered form of the encoded protein is produced by that allele. Normally, the protein made by the remaining normal allele is sufficient to keep the cell going, even if the mutant gene is completely functionless. But on occasion, the altered protein made by the mutant allele may interfere with the function of the normal protein produced by the unmutated allele within the same cell; the effect of the mutation "dominates" and negates the function of the normal gene product. Such mutations (called *transdominant* mutations) are especially likely to involve genes encoding proteins that must interact with each other to form multiprotein (*multimeric*) struc-

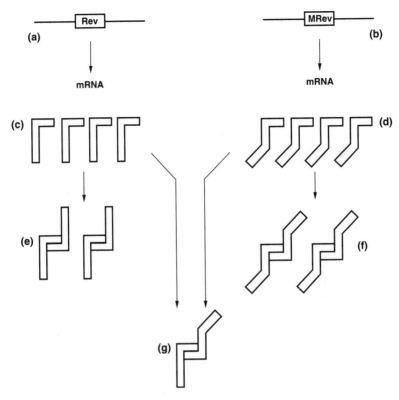

Figure 10-2. The dominant-negative strategy for interfering with HIV replication.
The Rev protein (c) aggregates into a multimeric structure (e) important in the HIV
replication cycle. A mutant Rev gene (b) encodes an altered form of this protein (d) that
still aggregates, but the resulting structure is conformationally distorted (f) and cannot
function. When the two genes are present in the same cell, the respective subunits can
aggregate, but the resulting structure (g) is sufficiently distorted that it cannot function
normally in HIV replication. By generating an excess of the mutant subunit in an HIV-
infected cell, production of normal Rev multimers can be essentially completely
suppressed.

tures. If one of the subunits (*monomers*) is shaped incorrectly, the function of the entire multimeric structure may be lost.

Gene therapy techniques could be used to deliver a transdominant
mutant form of a critical HIV gene into T cells or bone marrow. Specific
mutations are fairly easy to generate in the laboratory once a cloned copy
of the normal form of the gene is in hand, and the exact nucleotide
sequence for the gene is known. If the transdominant gene is delivered in
a retroviral vector, it will integrate into the targeted cell's DNA and act as

one allele for that particular gene. If the cell thus transduced is never infected by HIV, the presence of the transdominant HIV gene will cause neither harm nor benefit; the protein would be produced, but having no function it would just be continually synthesized, degraded, and replaced. But if such a transduced cell were to become infected with HIV, the virus would in effect provide a second, normal allele of the same protein. Both "alleles" would now make their proteins; if these proteins are used to build a multimeric protein structure, both allelic forms will be used. The transdominant mutant would render the resulting complexes useless for viral assembly, and viral replication would be greatly inhibited or stop. To enhance the effect of the transdominant gene, it can be equipped with a promoter that makes its production more efficient than its normal HIV counterpart, resulting in multimeric complexes that are predominantly composed of the mutant subunits.

This strategy has been used successfully to block HIV replication in human CD4 T cells grown in vitro. Again, the Rev gene is a good target. Like all proteins, Rev is made as a monomeric protein chain but, in order to carry out its function in escorting HIV mRNA out of the nucleus, it must first assemble itself into a multimeric structure. There is a stretch of amino acids at one end of each monomeric Rev chain that is essential in forming proper multimers. By altering the nucleotides in a normal Rev gene that code for these amino acids, mutant alleles of this "association region" can be generated that still allow multimers to form, but the resulting multimers cannot function to transport HIV mRNA. Experiments have shown that if even one of the monomers in a multimeric structure is mutant, the multimer will not function. Thus even a moderate number of mutant proteins can wreak havoc on HIV reproduction in a cell.

When human CD4 T cells were transduced with such transdominant mutant Rev genes, the transduced cells were able to be infected by HIV, and HIV proviral DNA was able to insert into the cells' DNA. The proviral DNA was apparently transcribed into mRNA for the various HIV proteins, but the mRNAs never made it out of the nucleus for translation, and no virus was produced by the infected cells. The Rev complex made from normal HIV Rev subunits, plus the transdominant mutant subunits, was not functional. On the other hand, the presence of the mutant Rev gene did not seem to interfere with normal CD4 T cell functions.

This approach to treating AIDS has now been approved for Phase I clinical trials at the University of Michigan, and the first patients have just been entered into these trials. In initial results published in April 1996, it was reported that CD4 T cells, removed from patients with early-stage AIDS, transduced in vitro with transdominant mutant Rev genes, and then reinfused into the same patient, showed dramatically prolonged survival compared with CD4 T cells transduced with a control gene. There were no adverse effects on the patients, and further studies are in progress to increase the efficacy of this treatment.

The dominant-negative strategy using Rev has also been incorporated into the NIH TAR antisense study described earlier. Some of the patients in the NIH study will have their CD4 T cells transduced with a TAR antisense gene alone, and some will have their cells transduced with a vector containing both a TAR antisense sequence and a transdominant Rev mutant gene. As long as each gene is under control of a functional promoter, there is no reason why a vector cannot be used to deliver two proteins instead of one. Each gene will integrate as part of the proviral DNA, and each will be transcribed into an RNA molecule. For the Rev transgene, this will be an mRNA that is translated into the mutant Rev protein. The TAR RNA will lack a start codon, and will not be translatable; it will function in its RNA form to block the TAR promoter sequence. Such double-barreled transgene approaches should be particularly effective in blocking HIV reproduction in cells.

Intracellular Immunization

The idea of embedding something inside a cell that would interfere with viral assembly or viral function (without affecting the cell's ability to carry out its own crucial tasks) has been carried a few steps further. Antibodies to viruses work well outside cells, where viruses are traveling in the bloodstream or lymph, but cannot get at viruses hiding inside cells. But what if the *gene* for a virus-specific antibody were introduced into a cell's DNA, so that the antibody was actually produced right there inside the virus-infected cell? This is one form of the approach called *intracellular immunization*. Genes encoding antibodies that can specifically recognize and bind to several different HIV proteins have been introduced into human CD4 T cells in the laboratory. In the absence of virus, the antibodies are made at a slow but steady rate, and like other unused proteins are disposed of by the cell through normal processes. But when these cells were subsequently infected by HIV, the targeted proteins were trapped by the waiting antibody molecules, and could not be used for viral assembly and function. The production of infectious HIV particles by these cells plummeted dramatically. The complexes of antibody and viral proteins were destroyed by the cell in a manner similar to the fate of the mutant protein complexes in dominant-negative experiments.

In a variation of this approach, T cells were transduced with the CD4 gene, modified so that its protein product would stay inside the cell rather than insert into the cell membrane. When such cells were infected with HIV, the gp120 protein made by the virus became ensnared by the intracellular CD4 molecules; the CD4 molecule in this case behaved just like an antibody would, and again the production of virus was greatly diminished.

For a variety of technical reasons, intracellular immunization strategies are not yet ready for the clinic, but they are exemplary of the imagination and insight that basic science is bringing to bear on the obliteration of this terrible disease. It is entirely possible that some version of this approach will make its way to the clinic in the next few years.

Suicide Revisited

The suicide-gene strategy proposed for use in cancer gene therapy may have AIDS applications as well. So far this approach has only been tested on human CD4 cells in the laboratory, but the results look highly promising and one or more variants of this technique may well move to the clinic in the near future. The way the suicide-gene strategy works is shown in Figure 10-3. When HIV proviral DNA begins to be expressed in infected CD4 cells, the viral genes are read in two phases. The first set of genes to be transcribed and translated are the so-called *regulatory genes*. The protein products of these genes (such as the Tat gene) interact with the promoter regions of the *structural genes* of the virus—the genes that encode the proteins needed for the construction of new viral particles.

The suicide approach to treating HIV-infected cells takes advantage of this carefully orchestrated expression of HIV genes. In a study carried out in a French research laboratory, human CD4 T cells were first transduced with an Hstk gene in a retroviral delivery vector similar to those used for treating cancer patients. However, in this vector the Hstk gene was placed under control of the same Tat-responsive promoter that regulates expression of the HIV structural genes. In the absence of HIV infection, the

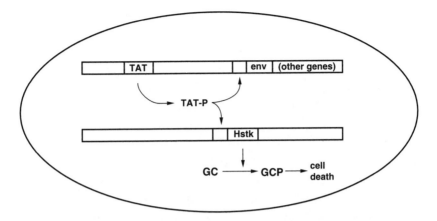

Figure 10-3. The suicide strategy for treating AIDS. The first step in viral reproduction is production of the TAT protein (TAT-P), which then activates env and other HIV genes. If the cell has previously been transduced with an Hstk gene under a TAT-requiring promoter, TAT-P will also activate the Hstk gene (even on another chromosome), which leads to the production of GCP if gancyclovir is present (see Figure 9-3). The HIV-infected cell will thus die, depriving the virus of a place to replicate.

Hstk gene in transduced cells will not be read, because the regulatory protein required to activate its promoter, Tat, is not present in uninfected cells. The cells were then exposed to HIV, and grown in an acyclovir medium. As the proviral genes began to express themselves in the infected cells, the Tat regulatory genes began to turn on not only the HIV structural proteins, but the Hstk genes as well. The HIV-infected cells promptly died from the acyclovir before they could produce new HIV particles. At levels of acyclovir normally found in patients treated with this drug for viral infections, the CD4 cells could be maintained in culture completely free of HIV.

In another variant of the suicide strategy, the gene for diphtheria toxin (DTα) was introduced into T cells under control of a Tat-activated promoter. DTα is one of the most deadly bacterial toxins known to humankind; a single molecule is enough to kill a cell. When T cells with the DTα gene were infected by HIV and Tat activated the DTα promoter, the cells died almost instantly. This rapid death prevented the production and release of infectious virus, as well as the release of poisonous DTα. The fear that DTα could harm surrounding normal cells in the body is a natural concern about using this particular approach in the clinic. However, the amounts involved could probably be handled by anyone with normal immunity to diphtheria, and further precautionary strategies to ensure that toxin production is kept under strict control in uninfected cells may yet allow this approach to make its way to the clinic.

All of the foregoing strategies to treat AIDS target the mature T cell. As was learned in the ADA-SCID trials involving mature T cell transduction, the numbers of altered T cells appearing in the circulation after reinfusion is initially rather low. Over time, those mature T cells that are rescued by gene therapy, and subsequently activated by antigen, will accumulate as memory cells and come to dominate in the overall population. But most of the T cells transduced by the delivery vector will turn over in the blood without ever being activated; the process of T-cell buildup over time may work too slowly to help a patient with active AIDS. On the other hand, this kind of treatment could work very well for someone with HIV infection who is still asymptomatic—the average time from HIV infection to onset of active disease is eight to ten years. Untransduced T cells infected by HIV will rapidly disappear from the circulation; T cells with an antisense "time bomb" planted inside would have a powerful survival advantage, and should come to dominate the T-cell compartment in short order. Also, it should theoretically be possible to introduce genes into the bone-marrow stem cells of AIDS patients using crippled forms of HIV itself as the vector. It will be ironic indeed if AIDS turns out to be treatable using an altered form of the very pathogen that causes it in the first place!

For AIDS, given that no current treatment is still more than marginally effective, gene therapy offers one of the brightest hopes on the treatment horizon. Unlike other current treatment methods, gene therapy has the potential to provide a cure for this disease. As a blood-cell disorder, delivery of protective genes should be relatively easy. And unlike the situation with cancer, in AIDS it will not be necessary to destroy every HIV-infected cell in the body to ameliorate the disease. If even a small proportion of T cells can be rescued—either in their mature form or as they are formed in the bone marrow—there is good reason to believe reasonably normal immune function could be restored.

The potential for AIDS to cause serious damage to the human species as a whole cannot be underestimated. If HIV ever mutates to a form that can be spread by something as simple as sneezing or shaking hands, it could wipe out major sections of the human population. Eventually it, too, would probably learn to live with its new host—us—in some sort of natural equilibrium. But we cannot afford to wait for a possible modus vivendi to develop, losing perhaps ninety percent of the human race in the process. As best we can tell, this most deadly of human diseases is with us in the first place because of our tendency to meddle with nature, invading its domains and driving pathogens from their normal hosts into our own bodies. But it just may be that HIV will ultimately fall victim to precisely that same predilection: our tendency, come to full flower in the research laboratory, to meddle with nature at its most fundamental level, the level of DNA itself.

11

Naked DNA

The Vaccine of the Future

Vaccination as it is currently practiced was introduced at the end of the eighteenth century by the English physician Edward Jenner. It involves the administration of minute amounts of a pathogen—a bacterium, virus, fungus, or occasionally a parasite—in one or more doses. The pathogen is either dead or attenuated (alive, but rendered unable to cause disease) but is still recognized by the immune system as foreign. Sometimes a fragment of the pathogen, or even a single molecule from the pathogen, will suffice for immunization because these, too, are recognized as foreign. The immune system then mounts a response against the pathogen or its components that is as effective as if the person thus immunized had been exposed to a fully active pathogen. Depending on the pathogen and how it is administered, protection may be long lasting or require periodic reexposure ("booster shots").

When Jenner first developed his technique, he had no idea what a "pathogen" really was. The work of Louis Pasteur, Robert Koch and others in the second half of the nineteenth century demonstrated that many diseases are caused by microorganisms (bacteria, viruses, funguses, and parasites) and that these are the diseases against which vaccination can provide protection. Vaccination has been extraordinarily effective in reducing illness and death stemming from infectious disease, particularly in children. In the case of one particularly deadly disease—smallpox, the malady against which Jenner's pioneering efforts were directed—a world-wide vaccination campaign administered through the World Health Organization led to its complete eradication in 1979. Similar campaigns mounted against polio and measles are expected to lead to the total elimination of these diseases shortly after the turn of the next century.

In spite of these impressive contributions to world health, vaccination is far from perfect. Effective vaccines are available for only a relatively small proportion of the infectious diseases that afflict humans. In some cases this lack of availability is simply a question of economics; vaccines can be very expensive to produce, and they may have a rather limited life-time. Their production only becomes feasible when they can be made in large quantities that are distributed and used quickly. In a few cases—cholera, for example—there is a huge potential market, but attempts to prepare an immunogenic form of the pathogen simply have succeeded only marginally in spite of years of effort.

Another shortcoming of vaccination generally is that it elicits almost exclusively an antibody response. Antibodies provide excellent protection against bacteria, which are responsible for a great many infectious diseases, but antibodies are only partially effective against many viruses. The major reason for this is that in our bodies viruses spend most of their time inside cells. Once a virus penetrates a cell and takes up residence there, it cannot be detected by antibodies. That is the job of "killer T cells," also known as cytotoxic T lymphocytes (CTL). These cells examine the surfaces of all other cells in the body. Fragments of proteins currently being produced inside a cell are displayed at its surface in a form recognized by CTL. If foreign proteins are produced inside a cell, for example by a virus replicating therein, CTL will destroy that cell.

Unfortunately, CTL responses are rarely if ever induced during the course of standard vaccination procedures. The material used for immunization purposes is either dead or disabled; the viruses used in vaccines are thus unable to infect a living cell. Since they cannot direct the synthesis of proteins inside a cell, CTL have no way of knowing they are in the body, and never become activated. Immunization with a killed virus or its components will of course induce the formation of antibodies. When the body is subsequently infected with a healthy virus, the antibodies may "pick off" the virus on its way to or from a cell (which is why antibodies may be partially effective against some viral infections). But once the new invader has reached a cell and taken up residence there, it is unreachable by antibody.

When a killed or attenuated pathogen used in standard vaccine materials first enters the body, it is immediately broken up by macrophages into its component molecules and fragments thereof, and it is these—rather than the intact pathogen itself—toward which the antibody response is directed. Quite often, particularly in the case of viruses, the entire antibody response may be directed to only one or a very few molecules or molecular fragments from the pathogen. That is why vaccination may occasionally be carried out with individual molecules isolated from the pathogen, if these are the molecular components known to induce immunity. Prominent among these components are proteins. But isolating highly purified protein samples from pathogens for use in vaccines is extremely time consuming and expensive. On the other hand, we know very well that proteins are produced in response to instructions from genes. Instead of trying to put an immunogenic protein itself into an individual in order to induce a protective immune response, why not simply introduce the gene encoding that protein? This thought is likely to revolutionize vaccination in the twenty-first century.

The process is as follows. A gene encoding a known immunogenic protein from a given pathogen is inserted into an appropriate delivery vector, and introduced into the body. The site doesn't matter; intramuscular injection works very well. The DNA will penetrate cells at the site of injection, and begin making the corresponding protein. The gene can be engineered to produce a protein that is released from the cell into the bloodstream, where it is picked up by macrophages and B cells, resulting in antibody production. But because the protein is actually synthesized within a cell in response to an internalized gene, fragments of the protein will also be displayed at the cell surface, triggering a CTL response as well. This is a tremendous advantage over standard immunization techniques that produce only an antibody response.

Because the immune system is so sensitive, it is not necessary to transduce large numbers of cells in vivo; the inefficiency of transduction that is so limiting in some gene therapy applications is not a problem here. In fact, researchers have found that it is not even necessary to use a special viral delivery vector; simple injection of the gene alone (so-called "naked DNA") works quite well. Cells such as those found in muscle tissue or skin take up enough DNA spontaneously to allow induction of a vigorous immune response to the corresponding protein. Even less DNA is required with a device called a "gene gun." Tiny amounts of DNA are coated onto microscopic gold beads, which are then shot under high pressure into the skin. As the beads pass through the outer layers of the skin, the DNA is in effect scraped off and taken up by surrounding cells. This technique can also be used to deliver DNA to deeper tissues in the body that have been exposed surgically, and may eventually find application for DNA delivery in standard gene therapy.

Whether it is actually skin and muscle cells per se that pick up the DNA is not clear. It could well be other cells such as macrophages or macro-phage-like dendritic cells that are known to be resident in these tissues. But that doesn't really matter; for vaccination purposes it is ultimately the immune system as a whole that is being targeted.

Muscle cells seem to be particularly adept at taking up injected DNA and incorporating it into their own nuclear DNA. This was a considerable surprise. Scientists would like to understand why this is so, what it is about muscle cells that is different from other cells. This could help them improve the entire DNA vaccination process. But it might also provide clues about getting naked DNA into cells other than muscle for general gene therapy purposes. Moreover, in those cases where the genetic defect is for production of a protein needed by the body generally, it might be possible to simply introduce the gene into muscle or skin, from where the corresponding protein could be released into the general circulation.

Some of the most striking preclinical results with this new approach to vaccination have been obtained in mice with the hepatitis B virus (HBV). HBV-induced hepatitis (sometimes also called serum hepatitis) afflicts over 300 million people worldwide, and is one of the leading causes of death from infectious disease. Vaccines are currently available, but they are expensive to produce and distribute, and have had little impact on hepatitis B outside the industrialized world (where most of the cases in fact arise). HBV causes both an acute and a chronic form of hepatitis, and is also a leading cause of liver cancer. In the acute form of the disease, the response by T cells, particularly CTL, is prompt and vigorous; through a combination of T cells and antibodies, the infection is rapidly cleared, although often with considerable liver damage. Antibodies eliminate viruses passing through the bloodstream, and CTL destroy virally infected cells. But in a certain number of cases, the immune response is not vigorous enough, and the infection becomes chronic. CTL continue to destroy HBV-infected cells, but never vigorously enough to clear the infection. Eventually, the accumulated liver damage continues to mount to a point where it cannot be repaired, and death from massive cirrhosis or progression into liver cancer is not uncommon. The consensus has been that if the initial T cell response were more vigorous, disease would be arrested at the acute stage, with moderate but acceptable (and repairable) liver damage.

In an attempt to bolster the CTL response in vivo, a strain of mice susceptible to the same HBV that infects humans was immunized with the gene encoding the major coat protein of this virus. The gene was first modified so that it could be cloned in a bacterial plasmid system, and placed under control of a strong promoter that works well in mammalian cells. The entire recombinant plasmid was isolated and used without further modification for direct intramuscular injection into susceptible mice. (The bacterial plasmid is unable to replicate in humans and poses no health risk in itself.) A few days later the mice were injected with a strong dose of HBV. They were extraordinarily resistant to this virus. Most importantly, CTL taken from these mice were able to kill HBV-infected cells in vitro, and produced inflammatory cytokines of the type that would bolster immune reponses in vivo. An antibody response was also induced, and was in fact much stronger than could be obtained by injecting the coat protein itself. Both the antibody and CTL response lasted many months.

One of the great hopes for vaccines of this type is that they may be effective even after an infection has set in. Current HBV vaccines induce a protective antibody response that can prevent infection in the first place. But in those cases where infection has already occurred, and has progressed to a chronic stage, it may still be possible to boost the CTL response with a DNA vaccine, thus ending the infection. DNA vaccines for HBV have now been tested in chimpanzees, in whom the course of HBV infection is virtually identical to humans. The results were excellent; human clinical trials with this vaccine are planned for the very near future.

Another highly promising application for DNA vaccines is in the prevention of tuberculosis, which kills more than three million people worldwide each year. The causative agent in tuberculosis is a bacterium rather than a virus, but because the tuberculosis bacterium actually takes up residence inside living cells (unusual for a bacterium), the immune response is the same, involving both antibodies and T cells, as well as macrophages. In this disease, both CTL and helper T cells are involved: the helper T cells are important in generating an unusually powerful inflammatory response, called a delayed-type hypersensitivity (DTH) reaction. This reaction is highly effective in eliminating infected cells. As with hepatitis B in the liver, most of the serious damage in chronic tuberculosis is caused by T cells trying to destroy infected lung cells, rather than by the bacterium itself, and the history of the disease within the body is also similar. If the early T cell response is strong enough, the bacterial infection is overcome, or at least stabilized. It is only when the infection becomes chronic as a result of an ineffective initial response that lung destruction reaches morbid or even lethal levels.

Once thought to be near extinction, TB is again on the rise in large urban centers around the world. Particularly deadly forms have arisen in immunocompromised individuals, such as those with AIDS, or patients being treated with immunosuppressive drugs in connection with organ transplantation. These new strains appear to be more aggressive and resistant to standard treatments. The standard vaccine for tuberculosis, which induces only an antibody response, was important in bringing tuberculosis under control early in this century. But there have always been individuals in whom the vaccine did not seem to work well. Moreover, the vaccines used are only attenuated, not killed; when introduced into an immunocompromised individual, the vaccine can, on occasion, cause disease. It is also not clear how effective current vaccines are against the newer, more aggressive strains of tuberculosis. For these and other reasons, infectious disease specialists have begun experimenting with DNA vaccines, particularly in an attempt to achieve an early and vigorous CTL response. Again using a mouse model, it has been found that exposure to several tuberculosis bacterial genes induced a strong protective response that involved antibodies, helper T cells, and, most importantly, CTL. This vaccine, too, is clearly headed for clinical trials in the not-too-distant future, and could be extremely valuable in once again bringing this dreaded disease under control.

DNA vaccines are now being actively explored for a wide range of infectious pathogens, including the ever-elusive influenza virus. Influenza virus, like HIV, has the unfortunate (for us) property of rapidly mutating its coat proteins. Since antibodies can only react with these outer coat proteins on a virus (they have no way of burrowing into the interior of the virus, just as they have no way of getting inside a cell), the antibodies produced in response to infection with one strain of flu have no protective effect a year or so later, when the flu virus has once again changed its coat. That is why there has never been an effective general vaccine for the flu. Enhancement of the CTL response to the internal proteins of the virus, which do not change from season to season, will not likely prevent us from getting the flu in the first place. It takes several days for a CTL response to get underway, and our immune systems are usually mobilized by then in direct response to the active infection. But, as with hepatitis, in those cases where we fail to clear the influenza virus rapidly enough on our own, or in immunocompromised individuals where a simple flu infection may progress into something much more deadly (ten to twenty thousand deaths are attributed to complications of influenza each year), induction of a strong CTL response with a vaccine may be very important indeed.

DNA vaccination could be particularly important for extremely dangerous viruses such as Ebola or Marburg. These pathogens spread very rapidly from person to person, and can cause a fatal hemorrhagic fever in as little as forty-eight hours. So far these viruses—for which the natural host is unknown—have only infected humans at a few sites on the sub-Saharan African continent. The ensuing morbidity and mortality is so rapid that, together with quick recognition and rapid action by local health authorities, these outbreaks have been fairly well contained.

But what would happen if a recently infected person stepped on an airplane bound for a major human population center, where local officials might not immediately recognize the ensuing symptoms, and the infection began to spread? Arriving in an airport, an infected individual could transmit the virus in aerosol form to persons about to board airplanes to yet other cities. Huge numbers of people in many different locations would have to be immunized, and very quickly. Large-scale preparation of killed forms of these viruses, or of their component proteins, is simply out of the question; they are far to dangerous to handle in an industrial setting. Fortunately, both viruses have been grown and dissected at sites such as the Centers for Disease Control in Atlanta, and the Army's Infectious Disease Center at Frederick, Maryland. All of the genes important for a vaccine have been isolated and cloned. Stocks of these genes could be scaled up in a matter of days, and shipped to affected areas for immediate use. Given that the forms of these viruses infecting humans have not yet shown up in the Western Hemisphere, mass preventative vaccination programs could not be justified, but based on the experience in Africa, we would do well to be prepared to move quickly.

A form of DNA vaccination may even have a role to play in cancer. As we know, many tumors are inherently immunogenic, but for various reasons fail to induce a sufficiently strong immune response. In some cases, the antigens on a tumor to which the body could potentially respond are known, and the genes encoding these molecules have actually been isolated and cloned. Several laboratories are now investigating the possibility of introducing these "tumor antigens" into the body in the form of a DNA vaccine. One such study, which has already reached the stage of testing in chimpanzees, involves the MUC-1 gene. MUC-1 is expressed on many tumors of epithelial cell origin (*carcinomas*) arising in tissues as diverse as lung, colon, breast, and pancreas. Since MUC-1 is produced as an internal protein, it is puzzling that a strong CTL response is not generated. Part of the reason may be that tumor cells are not themselves very effective presenters of internally produced proteins. Recently, the MUC-1 gene was introduced into radiated chimpanzee cells that were known to be effective in this form of antigen presentation. The altered cells were then returned to the animals. Over the next several weeks, a very strong CTL response to MUC-1 was noted; the chimps showed no untoward effects from the procedure.

DNA vaccination has the potential to greatly improve and extend the benefits of immunization as currently practiced. Even developing countries have the technical expertise to carry out such procedures; since DNA is very stable, vaccines and vaccine mixtures can be prepared, distributed, and stored for long periods of time if necessary. Moreover, one can use a mixture of different genes from a given pathogen in the same immunization procedure, greatly increasing the efficiency of immunization against pathogens whose immunogenic components are not precisely known. It is also possible to combine genes from several pathogens in the same vaccine. Vaccines for pathogens such as Ebola and Marburg could well be used prophylactically in at least parts of Africa. Perhaps most important of all is the reduced cost of DNA vaccines. It seem highly likely that the DNA vaccine for HBV described earlier—which combines the antibody-producing effectiveness of exisiting vaccines, with a strong CTL response, all at a greatly reduced cost—will soon be available for use worldwide. This vaccine, and others like it that will surely follow, will have a profound effect on human health in the twenty-first century.

12

The Human Genome Project

By the end of the 1980s, the approximate chromosomal locations were known for nearly two thousand human genes, and partial or complete nucleotide sequences were in hand for about 500; the two groups only partially overlapped. But progress in identifying, cloning, and sequencing new human genes was definitely slowing down. Many of the first human genes to be cloned and sequenced had been relatively "easy." In some cases, the protein sequence was already known, allowing synthesis of a corresponding DNA probe for locating the gene on a southern blot. In other cases, a gene cloned from an animal source could be used as a probe to find its human counterpart. But increasingly, human gene sequences were obtained only at the end of long, tedious, expensive, and highly focused searches related to specific human diseases—the CFTR gene was a case in point. The value of knowing the sequence of the CFTR gene is obvious: more precise genetic screening; an unambiguous protein sequence for studying the metabolic basis of the CF defect; the possibilities of gene replacement therapy. But given the very large number of human genetic diseases, it is equally obvious that this type of ad hoc approach to gene isolation and sequencing is too inefficient if molecular medicine is to have a meaningful impact on human health. It was this realization that ultimately gave birth to the Human Genome Project.

The Human Genome Project (HGP) approaches the problems of gene identification and sequencing from a completely different perspective; it reverses their order. It abandons ad hoc isolation and sequencing of individual genes on a disease-by-disease basis in favor of systematic sequencing of the entire human genome. The expense and labor of tracing the location and establishing the identification of individual genes (by far the most costly and time-consuming parts of the overall process in the past) are largely set aside until the human genome has been sequenced in its entirety. Once this database has been established, it will serve as a comprehensive listing as well as a map for locating and retrieving all human genes.

The data already obtained from sequencing the genomes of microorganisms suggests that completion of HGP will result in a veritable treasure trove of new genetic information about humans. It will greatly accelerate the identification of the several thousand remaining disease genes. We will of course in the process also identify the 90,000-plus genes *not* associated with disease—although many may turn out to have previously unsuspected disease associations. We will doubtless uncover the traces of thousands of retroviral-type viruses that have burrowed their way into the human genome over millions of years. We will also gain a new understanding of the nucleotide changes (mutations) that can occur in our genes without giving rise to disease. And we will almost certainly come across genes we did not even know existed. We will, after all, have before us a detailed diagram of all the genes necessary to direct the construction and operation of an entire human being. Ultimately we will want to understand the function of every one of those genes. When we do, we will understand a great deal more about ourselves as biological organisms than we ever have before.

The Human Genome Project may well turn out to be one of the most expensive, highly focused undertakings in the history of biomedical science, the biologist's equivalent of sending a man to the moon. Initial cost estimates were in the range of three billion dollars over a fifteen-year period; we may actually do it in slightly less time, for slightly less money.

But *why* are we doing it? Will the information gained at the end justify the diversion of so many human and financial resources for such a long period of time? Whose idea was this, anyway?

How It All Began

The nucleotide sequence for the first human gene—the gene for the red blood cell protein b-globin—was published in 1977. This did not catch anyone by surprise. By the mid-1970s, molecular biologists all over the world were in the race to apply their rapidly developing technologies— applied so successfully to the sequencing of viral and bacterial genes—to the isolation and sequencing of human genes. Partial sequences of literally dozens of other human genes were already in the pipeline, and would also be published over the next few years. It is possible to obtain the sequence for a gene without knowing its chromosomal location, and it is possible to know the chromosomal location for a gene without knowing anything about its sequence. Both activities—chromosomal mapping and gene sequencing—continued at a frantic pace throughout the 1970s and 1980s, but it was precisely these activities that began to slow so markedly as the 1980s drew to a close.

No one person in particular is credited with being the first to think of mapping and sequencing the entire human genome, three billion base pairs containing all one hundred thousand human genes in the complete set of human chromosomes. The genomes for two viruses—many orders of magnitude smaller than mammalian genomes—had been completed already in 1975 and 1976. One imagines that the idea of sequencing the human genome must have flitted at one time or another through the mind of anyone working on human DNA cloning and sequencing. The possibility of such an undertaking was discussed with varying degrees of seriousness at scientific meetings—at first mostly in hotel lobbies after hours, or over hurried meals between daytime plenary sessions and work-shops; later on in the working sessions themselves.

Several events taking place during the mid-1980s are generally cred-ited with stimulating large segments of the biomedical community to think in terms of a national-level, organized human genome project. One of these was a meeting in December 1984 at a ski resort in Alta, Utah, sponsored by the U.S. Department of Energy (DOE). As the direct lin-eal descendent of the original Manhattan Project and the former Atomic

Energy Commission, DOE had a long-standing interest in the effect of radiation on human DNA. One of their most venerable projects was (and continues to be) the analysis of the occurrence and transmission of genetic mutations in survivors of Hiroshima and Nagasaki. It had been realized for some years that many genotypic alterations (mutations) might have been induced in the DNA of these people that were not readily observable because they did not result in obvious phenotypes whose inheritance could be followed by standard genetics. What seems to have emerged from this meeting was the notion that the ideal way to quantitate all radiation damage to DNA, and either its repair or its transmission from one generation to the next, would be the direct comparison of very large stretches of DNA sequence between parents and offspring. Long-term survivors of these blasts by definition would be expected to have only minor DNA damage, and detection of this damage could require sequencing of substantial portions of their genome. This led to the first serious discussions of large-scale DNA sequencing in humans, and what it would entail.

The next event referred to by HGP historians (projects as massive and as costly as HGP tend to generate history and attract historians very quickly) was a meeting called the following year by the eminent molecular biologist-*cum*-university chancellor, Robert Sinsheimer. In May 1985 Sinsheimer invited a small but stellar group of research colleagues from the U.S. and abroad to his University of California campus at Santa Cruz. Sinsheimer was aggressively seeking a major scientific program in which his campus—the newest of the nine-member UC system—could participate and establish its reputation as a research center of the first rank. His scientific antennae had intercepted a good deal of recent chatter about a major genome effort, and his political instincts told him this could be exactly the project he was looking for.

DOE was clearly thinking along the same lines. Charles DeLisi, a physicist and director of one of the DOE's branches, was casting about for ways to redirect his agency as the world began to back away from nuclear self-destruction. The DOE had been supporting some of the emerging studies on DNA sequencing technology. In fact the agency had established, in 1983, the first large-scale registry of the many DNA sequences that were beginning to accumulate for organisms ranging from viruses to humans. (This registry, called GenBank, is to this day one of the primary resources for storage and retrieval of DNA sequence information worldwide.) Fol-lowing up on the Alta meeting of the year before, DeLisi called another DOE-sponsored meeting in March 1986, just ten months after Sins-heimer's exploratory session. This meeting took place at the Los Alamos National Laboratory, and was attended by some of the same scientists. The mood at both meetings was very upbeat; there was a strong feeling that the basic techniques for sequencing the human genome were in hand, and that the rapidly accelerating pace of techno-logical improvements would make such a project feasible in a reasonable amount of time, somewhere between ten and twenty years.

Within days of the Los Alamos meeting, Renato Dulbecco of the Salk Institute in La Jolla independently published an essay in a widely dis-tributed journal in which he called for a national effort to map and sequence the entire human genome as part of the war on cancer. Dulbecco, a physicist who became a Nobel Prize–winning molecular biol-ogist, is one of the most respected figures in the field, and his opinion carried commensurate weight. Finally, in June of the same year, the pres-tigious annual gathering of scientists at Cold Spring Harbor, New York, chose for its theme the not unambitious topic, "The Molecular Biology of *Homo sapiens*." The Cold Spring Harbor meetings are far from rump sessions of a few select individuals; over three hundred of the country's top molecular biologists (and budding gene therapists such as French Anderson) attended the meeting. At this meeting, the DOE announced that it was seriously entertaining the possibility of underwriting a human genome sequencing project. That certainly got everyone's attention.

The concept of a gigantic, federally funded Human Genome Project was not without its doubters and detractors. The main concern expressed was the cost, and the fear that the cost would be carved out of the exist-ing government commitment to supporting basic biomedical research. Which ongoing research projects would be reduced or cut off altogether in order to support genome research? The National Institutes of Health, which was funding the lion's share of biomedical research in the U.S., including genome-related projects already underway, was becoming increasingly nervous about the eagerness of DOE to move into genome research in a big way. Such a project would have enormous health impli-cations, which the NIH regarded as its turf. Moreover, the culture at the two agencies was very different. DOE, dominated by physical scientists, was used to big-science, high-cost, multicenter projects. The tradition at NIH was to fund a larger number of small, innovative, single-investigator grants. Most scientists in the NIH fold viewed the mechanical cranking out of a several-billion-nucleotide-long DNA sequence as frankly boring; the physicists found it a delightful technological challenge.

The final push toward a coordinated national effort to map and sequence the entire human genome came from two 1988 reports. The first, published by the Office of Technology Assessment (which, until its disestablishment in 1994, advised Congress on scientific matters), was prohibited from endorsing such a project outright, but made it clear that it would be feasible and would have many benefits. The second report was issued by the National Research Council (NRC), the branch of the National Academy of Sciences that advises federal agencies on science policy issues. A special committee, chaired by the highly respected molecular biologist Bruce Alberts of the University of California at San Francisco, had been appointed to examine whether, how and to what extent the U.S. government should involve itself in supporting a coordinated effort to explore the human genome. The NRC report came down tactfully but strongly and clearly on the side of such a project. Among their recommendations were the following:

• The U.S. government should support an effort to first map and then sequence the entire human genome. This effort should receive support in the range of $200,000,000 per year for fifteen years. This support should be from money specifically granted by Congress for this purpose, and should not be diverted from the current budgetary allocations for basic biomedical research.

• The overall genome project should also support sequencing of the genomes of organisms other than humans, because of the past proven value of information obtained in such systems for interpreting the basic biology of human beings.

• A portion of the funding should be directed toward the development of existing or new technologies to increase the speed with which such a project could be carried out.

• A federal office should be created to coordinate the Human Genome Project, and to compile and help interpret the data collected by investigators around the country.

In December 1987, Congress appropriated funds to plan for and then establish genome projects at both the NIH and DOE, with the NIH getting the lion's share. The following year, James Wyngaarden, the then-director of NIH, established the Center for Human Genome Research as a permanent NIH Division. James Watson, of Watson-and-Crick fame, was named its first director. DOE had actually already created its own Human Genome Program the year before, with Benjamin Barnhart as its first director. The two agencies signed a memorandum of understanding in the fall of 1988. It was agreed that, in general, NIH would concentrate mainly on gene mapping, while DOE would focus mostly on DNA sequencing and its allied technologies, with the understanding that there might well be overlap in the two missions. A number of senior political and scientific leaders expressed concern about a wide range of anticipated ethical issues inherent in the Human Genome Project. Accordingly, both NIH and DOE pledged that a portion of the funds allocated to HGP through NIH would be targeted to an exploration of associated ethical issues.

Mapping the Human Genome

The first goal of HGP is to generate a complete map of the human genome, to guide scientists as they seek out specific genes in the future. A genome map is akin to an index for the six thousand or so volumes our DNA manuscripts will fill; it will tell us where in the genome the various genes can be found, and is preparatory to the actual retrieval, sequencing, and therapeutic use of individual genes. Genome maps can be of two types: genetic and physical. HGP will produce both, and then merge them into a single definitive human genome map. The object of genetic mapping is to assign genes or other genetic markers to individual chromosomes, and to *relative* positions on those chromosomes. This was the work begun just after the turn of the century when Morgan and Sturtevant began ordering the genes along the *Drosophila* X chromosome. The object of physical mapping is to generate physical fragments of the various chromosomes, to determine the order of the fragments along the chromosomes, and then to associate with each of them specific genes or markers pulled from the genetic map. Such fragments would ultimately serve as starting material for DNA sequencing.

The first human gene was mapped to an autosome only in 1968. At the time HGP got underway, the chromosomal locations for only about one percent of the estimated 100,000 human genes had been determined.

The techniques used up to that point were largely classical methods: inheritance studies plus somatic cell genetics, coupled with standard molecular biology of the time. As we saw with the mapping and identification of the CF gene, these are powerful tools indeed. But such procedures are not nearly powerful enough for the goals of HGP. One of the things that made HGP feasible was that by the mid-1980s, molecular biologists had devised completely new ways of mapping the genome. One of these procedures, as crucial to large-scale genome mapping as restriction nucleases were to gene cloning, involves something called *restriction fragment length polymorhisms* (RFLPs, or "riflips" for short). RFLPs were first proposed for mapping purposes in a paper published in 1980 by David Botstein, Ray White, Mark Skolnick, and Ron Davis, based on discussions they had had at another Alta meeting in 1978. By 1982, the method was in full swing in laboratories around the world. We have already encountered RFLPs, without identifying them as such, when we talked about the genetic markers MET and D7S8 in connection with CF. Without these markers, isolation of the CF gene would almost certainly have taken several years more to complete. As we will see in Chapter 13, RFLPs are also used in identifying biological samples, and often play a critical role in criminal trials.

The concept of a RFLP is fundamental to a great many of the applications of molecular biology to human biology and human health, and is illustrated in Figure 12-1. Classical gene mapping is based on the inheritance of mutated genes. A mutated gene, in reality, is nothing more than an allele of a given gene; it is "mutant" only because that particular allele functions in some observable way that is different from "normal" versions of the gene. It may cause wrinkled peas, or white eyes, or SCID. In classical genetics, the differences caused by mutated genes are traced in breeding experiments, and by establishing and refining exactly which chromosomes and which portions of chromosomes are inherited along with the various mutant properties. Over time, the genes involved are mapped to smaller and smaller regions of the genome.

Exactly the same thing is done with RFLPs, except one studies the inheritance of a RFLP rather than a gene. Most importantly, the inheritance of a RFLP is not followed by monitoring an associated phenotype; the RFLP itself is followed by direct examination of each generation's DNA. Identification of a RFLP begins with the isolation and cloning of a completely random "restriction fragment" of DNA. Such fragments (the

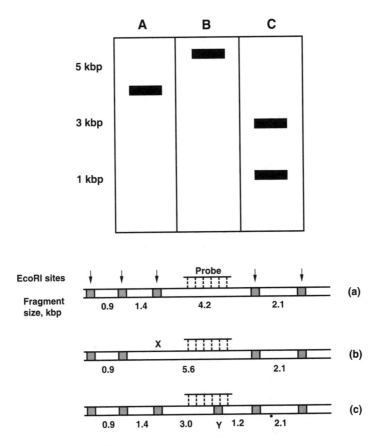

Figure 12-1. Restriction fragment length polymorphisms (RFLPs). The DNA from three different individuals (A-C) is cut with the same restriction enzyme, and subjected to Southern analysis (see Figure 5-3) using a probe generated from the DNA of one of the individuals (A). The probe shows a different pattern in each case, i.e., it detects a fragment of DNA that is of a different size in each individual's DNA. The origin of this size difference can be understood in terms of small nucleotide differences that affect the requisite cleavage motif for the enzyme. In individual B, one of the restriction sites present in A has been destroyed by a single nucleotide change (at "X"); the fragment detected by the probe is thus defined by the remaining downstream cleavage site, and the next upstream site, yielding a fragment of 5.6 kbp. In the case of individual C, a single nucleotide change ("Y") has created a new site within A's 4.2 kbp fragment, generating two smaller fragments that react with the probe.

"RF" in RFLP) are generated by digesting DNA with a particular restriction enzyme. The cloned DNA restriction fragment is then made radioactive or fluorescent and used as a probe for Southern blot analysis.

Let us assume that the DNA subjected to Southern analysis is from the same individual whose DNA was used to generate the probe, and that it is digested with the same restriction enzyme. As we saw earlier, the result of digestion and southern blotting will be a collection of DNA fragments of various sizes. Using the previously cloned fragment as a probe, we can ask what is the size (the length in nucleotides) of the restriction fragment reacted with by our cloned DNA fragment. Since the sample DNA is cut with the same restriction enzyme used to produce the cloned fragment we are using as a probe, then the probe is essentially reacting with itself. Suppose this probe is a fragment of, say, 4,200 base pairs, or 4.2 kbp, in the shorthand of molecular biologists. Then in this case it will detect a piece of DNA in the digested sample with a length (the "L" in RFLP) of 4.2 kbp on the Southern blot, since it is detecting itself (Figure 12-1a).

Suppose we now repeat this procedure using exactly the same probe, and exactly the same restriction enzyme, but using DNA samples collected from a large number of different individuals. Let us imagine that in such a random collection of individual DNA samples, our cloned probe reacts with three different sizes of fragments: some people have the 4.2 kbp fragment originally detected, others have a 5.0 kbp fragment, and still others show two fragments reacting with our probe—a 3.0 kb fragment, and a 1.2 kbp fragment. Our probe has defined a genetic *polymorphism* (the "P" in RFLP) in human DNA based on restriction fragment length; we have now defined a complete "riflip." This is the very essence of what RFLPs are all about. Just as human populations may have multiple forms of a regular gene, detected by different phenotypes, they may also have multiple forms of a RFLP. And just as there can be many different alleles of the same gene within a population, there can also be dozens or even hundreds of variants of the same RFLP in a population.

What is the origin of this polymorphism, and what is its significance? As shown in Figure 12-1a, the fragment of DNA detected by our cloned probe on the original southern blot has a length of 4.2 kbp because it lies between two restriction sites on a given chromosome separated by that many DNA nucleotides. When reacted with digested DNA from the same donor, that has been cut with the same enzyme, it detects a fragment identical in length to itself; it is detecting an exact copy of itself. But what happens if, in a portion of the human population, a nucleotide substitution has occurred at one of the restriction sites defining this fragment? This particular restriction site disappears; the restriction enzyme we are using no longer cuts there. However, our probe still does detect a fragment—in this case a fragment 5.6 kbp long (Figure 12-1b). This fragment is defined by the one remaining, unmodified restriction site for our enzyme, and the next restriction site upstream of the site destroyed by the nucleotide change. A different sized fragment can also be generated if a nucleotide substitution occurs within the previously defined fragment such that a new restriction site is created; the original 4.2 kb fragment is now split into two subfragments, each of which reacts with our probe (Figure 12-1c).

The important point is that the RFLPs we are defining by this procedure are, for the purposes of studying patterns of inheritance, *the functional equivalent of the alleles of genes found in populations*. If our original probe had not detected polymorphisms (varient alleles) of itself in the general population (and many probes would not), then it would not have been a RFLP, and would be of no use to us. Like alleles of true genes, RFLPs are based on nucleotide changes within a defined region of DNA. The only difference is that alleles of genes are normally defined by following observable characteristics (phenotypes) in breeding experiments; RFLPs are defined by size differences in DNA fragments identified by cloned probes, which are themselves restriction fragments. Thus RFLPs are followed in breeding experiments by direct examination of an offspring's DNA. Individuals of each of the three restriction fragment groups defined above will always transmit their own defined restriction fragment patterns for this probe to their offspring. The same probe can be used to detect this RFLP in their progeny. And that is the incredible power of the RFLP approach: we can generate millions of DNA fragments on our own that behave just as genes do, without having to actually associate them with any particular biological function.

But how are we any farther ahead by having functionless DNA fragments to play with? For one thing, we can physically map individual RFLPs to chromosomes rather precisely by a technique called *in situ hybridization*. If a restriction fragment or probe is made highly radioactive, and reacted with a set of chromosomes spread out on a glass microscope slide, the probe will bind tightly and specifically to its complementary DNA site on the chromosome; unbound probe can be washed away. If a piece of X-ray film is then placed over the spread chromosomes, a black dot will appear over the particular region of the specific chromosome to which the probe is bound. By correlating this position with the established banding pattern for this chromosome, a fairly specific location for the probe fragment can be defined.

But still, how does this help us locate human genes? To understand this, we have only to think back to Morgan and Sturtevant's concept of linkage groups. If we had a very large set of RFLPs for the human genome, such that we could define one RFLP for every million or so nucleotides along each chromosome, we could then ask a simple question: When we follow the phenotype of a disease-causing gene (or any other gene for that matter) in breeding experiments, which RFLPs always move together with the gene? To which RFLPs is our gene most tightly linked? Once we know that, we will then know precisely on which chromosome our gene is located, and to a fair degree of certainty, exactly where on that chromosome it is to be found.

The most useful RFLPs are in fact generally found in "nonsense" DNA, the ninety-five percent or so of the human genome that does not encode proteins. The nucleotide sequences for these regions (scattered more or less evenly throughout the genome) tend to vary a great deal among individuals. There is apparently no selective pressure operating to prevent nucleotide changes, and what in functional genes might be considered mutations, in noncoding DNA. A particularly useful type of RFLP is found in regions of the human genome characterized by enormous numbers of end-to-end repeats of three to five bp motifs, for example, $(ACAG)_n$, where n could be anywhere between fifty and one thousand. These *short tandem repeats* (STRs) are scattered throughout the genome, and many of them are highly polymorphic in the human population. What is polymorphic about STRs is not their nucleotide composition, but the *number* of repeats an individual may have. Different alleles are thus defined by size rather than by sequence. But that does not matter; these STRs and other RFLPs have proved invaluable in genetic mapping studies, and have also been extremely useful in identifying DNA specimens from individual human beings. (We will discuss such "forensic" uses of DNA technology in the next chapter.)

Genetic mapping of the human genome was essentially completed by the end of 1994, somewhat ahead of the time anticipated at the start of HGP. Using techniques similar to the RFLP approach, a French group (various European countries are involved in HGPs of their own, with a wide degree of cooperation with the U.S. effort) published a comprehensive map of identifiable genetic markers located on average about every 700,000 nucleotides throughout the entire human genome. Although eventually it may be useful to have a somewhat more detailed genetic map—with markers spaced perhaps no more than 250,000 nucleotides apart—the existing degree of resolution is sufficient to greatly speed the location and isolation of any human gene for which there is a mutation or a probe. Based on this map alone, a project such as that for isolating the CFTR gene could now be completed in a matter of months rather than years, and for a tenth the cost.

As can be appreciated from the way mapping is done, whether by following phenotypically observable mutations or RFLPs, if all human genomes were the same, we could not map them. Therefore, an important question associated with the mapping aspect of HGP is: Just whose genome are we sequencing, anyway? The answer is: Everyone's and no one's. There are literally billions of different human genomes; even the genomes of identical twins are not absolutely identical. But the differences, particularly in functional genes, are in fact quite minute, and that is what ultimately makes mapping and sequencing possible: we are all 99.9 percent or more identical. Scientists involved in HGP will be using pooled DNA that is as diverse as practical. Different laboratories will expect to find those occasional random nucleotide changes that give rise to mutations and RFLPs; their location and identity will be obvious through comparisons of DNA stretches sequenced in one laboratory with the same stretches sequenced in other labs. But the ability of a given defined DNA stretch to react with a specific probe will always provide the clue to its precise identity, even when it contains the occasional renegade nucleotide, connoting human diversity, within its sequence.

Physical Mapping of the Human Genome

The objective of physical mapping is to physically dissociate the genome into a collection of relatively small pieces, to "tag" each of them with a known marker, and then to order these pieces along the chromosomes much as the loci of genes or RFLPs are ordered on a genetic map. Rather than start with the entire human genome randomly cut up, most researchers begin with an individual chromosome or chromosomal frag-

197

ment that has been stably incorporated into an animal cell line carried in vitro (see section on somatic cell genetics, page 70.) As genes and RFLPs are identified and mapped genetically, they are ultimately associated with one and only one of these defined fragments, thus locating the genes or RFLPs physically in the DNA itself, as opposed to mapping them to a relative position on an entire chromosome. It will then be possible to recover a specific DNA fragment from the genome, and from that fragment to retrieve any of the genes known to be associated with it.

The obvious way to cut up the entire genome is with restriction enzymes. Unfortunately, most restriction enzymes create fragments that are too small to be practical, usually on the order of a few kbp. Given that the human genome contains approximately three billion base pairs, generation of three to four kbp fragments would produce around a million different fragments. Determining the location and order of that many fragments would be totally impractical. Recently, however, restriction enzymes have been found that generate fragments of between 100,000 and 1,000,000 nucleotides. This would reduce the total number of fragments to something like 10,000, which is generally considered to be doable.

Once the chromosomal fragments are generated from an initial DNA sample, they need to be cloned and expanded into large numbers of copies suitable for laboratory handling. Such fragments are much too large to be cloned into bacterial plasmids or even cosmids. The most useful way for cloning DNA fragments of this size is something called *yeast artificial chromosomes* (YACs). YACs had just been developed about the time HGP was coming under serious consideration (1986–7), and together with RFLPs was one of the technical advances that helped to convince the skeptics such a project could possibly succeed. Maynard Olson in St. Louis showed that portions of yeast chromosomes could be physically cut away, and replaced with defined chromosomal fragments from other species of up to several hundred thousand nucleotides. The newly incorporated material is reproduced normally when the yeast cell divides, and can be recovered after expansion of the yeast cell population in vitro. The basic idea is not all that different from plasmid cloning, except that the inserts are hundreds of times larger. Plasmids are epichromosomal genetic units that replicate in bacteria in synchrony with the bacterial cell chromosome. With YACs, the procedure has simply been moved up a notch in size: the much larger yeast cells replace the bacteria, and chromosomal fragments replace the plasmids. A similar technique using whole bacterial chromosomes as cloning vectors has produced the bacterial artificial chromosome (BAC), which hold slightly smaller DNA inserts (see Table 5-1).

As originally envisioned, a complete set of YAC clones containing human chromosome fragments would have been mapped and stored in a central human genome "library," and made available to anyone who needed them. For a variety of technical reasons, this approach has not quite worked out. One problem is that during the process of preparing human chromosomal fragments for insertion into YACs, many of the human fragments tend to stick together and form artificial "mosaic" chromosomal inserts. More than one fragment may end up in the same YAC, and the fragments would likely be from different chromosomes. While researchers can usually unravel this in the laboratory, in the long run it is bound to create confusion for those retrieving information from the library. A second problem is that the cost of maintaining a YAC library of the entire genome—especially if it has to be constantly checked for errors and mosaicism—turns out to be much higher than originally expected.

So rather than rely entirely on a single, common centralized bank of YAC clones covering the entire human genome, researchers have evolved another strategy called "sequence-tagged sites" (STSs.) STSs are conceptually similar to RFLPs, except that they rely not on polymorphic genes or DNA segments for their identity, but rather on sequences that are absolutely unique (i.e., occurring only once in the genome, and not varying from person to person). Such sequences often are associated with highly conserved portions of genes, although they need not be. The only requirement for STSs is that if the human genome is cut up into fragments of manageable size, each such fragment should be uniquely identifiable by one or more unique STSs. A central source of actual cloned fragments is then not necessary; it is the identity of the invariant STSs, and the specific chromosomal fragment they represent, that will be stored in a centralized data base. Anyone could then generate a collection of chromosomal fragments in their own laboratory using the appropriate restriction enzyme, and use the STS information to generate probes and isolate specific fragments in which they have an interest.

Association of individual genes, RFLPs, or STSs with specific YAC chromosomal fragments has been greatly aided by a powerful laboratory technique called *the polymerase chain reaction* (PCR). This method for finding DNA stretches for which the nucleotide sequence is known (or can be deduced from amino acid sequence data) has revolutionized molecular biology, in part because it is so sensitive it can accurately detect DNA sequences in as few as a dozen cells. The importance of this technique was recognized with the award of a Nobel Prize to its discoverer, Kary Mullis, in 1993.

The way PCR works is shown in Figure 12-2. A DNA sample is first *denatured* by heating, causing the two strands to separate from one another. Then a vast excess of PCR *primers* is added to the sample. Primers are akin to DNA probes in that they are short DNA stretches that match a portion of the gene or other sequence they are meant to detect. In fact, if PCR primers were made radioactive or fluorescent enough, they could be used as standard probes. But they can serve a much more interesting purpose. The primers are designed to attach to the targeted DNA sequence at either end, on opposite strands. Then, a special form of the enzyme DNA polymerase fills in the gap between the two primers with nucleotides. The reaction (which takes only a few minutes) is then stopped, and the entire mixture denatured once again. The original strands as well as the primers and the newly minted DNA products all separate, and the reaction mixture is cooled. Upon cooling, the original DNA strands and the new PCR products preferentially interact with more PCR primers rather than each other, because the primers are present in such great excess. The reaction is allowed to run again, and then the whole process is repeated over and over. The amount of PCR product (the short DNA stretch between the two primers) generated doubles at each round, whence the designation "chain reaction." Within a short time the PCR product—even starting from the tiny amount of DNA found in a single cell—will have been amplified sufficiently to be detected on a standard electrophoresis gel. Because the primers are absolutely specific for the DNA sequence in question, and because the precise distance between the primers is known in advance, the generation of a PCR product of the correct size is a highly reliable indication that the corresponding DNA sequence was present in the sample tested. PCR has been of value not only in the physical mapping of the human genome, but in genetic screening and in forensic applications as well.

PCR has been especially useful in assigning STSs to individual chromosomal fragments. The DNA sequence of PCR primers needed to iden-

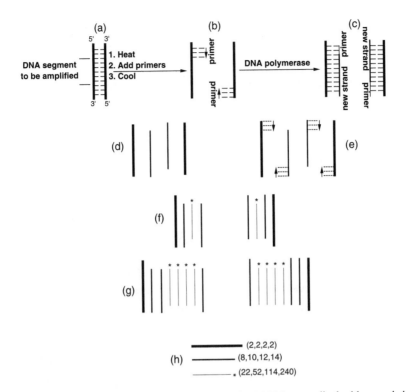

Figure 12-2. The polymerase chain reaction (PCR). DNA is normally double-stranded (a). When dsDNA is heated, the strands separate and primers flanking the region to be amplified associate with them (b). DNA polymerase fills in the the missing DNA sequences next to each primer (c), completing the first PCR cycle. No ligase is present to link the primer with the newly synthesized strand in each case. The products of the first cycle are the two original DNA strands, and two new strands that are somewhat shorter than the opposing original strands ("intermediate strands"; (d)). The reaction mixture is again heated; the four strands resulting from the first cycle separate separate, and associate with the excess primer remaining in the mixture (e). In this second PCR cycle, the left hand pair of strands (or chains) in (e) produces the four chains shown in the left half of (f); the right hand pair in (e) produces the chains shown on the right side of (f). (Both sets of reaction products are of course in the same tube.) Note here for the first time the appearance of the definitive PCR product (asterisk); this chain is exactly equal in length to the DNA bracketed by the primers in the original DNA sample. In the next cycle (g), this chain is just equal in number to the sum of the other two chains; with succeeding cycles, this chain will come to predominate. The original two strands remain in the mixture, but do not expand; the intermediate strands expand arithmetically, two more being generated at each round. The true PCR product expands geometrically (hence the name "chain reaction"), and after a dozen or so cycles the other chains are a negligible part of the overall composition of the product. The frequency of the original chains, the intermediate chains and the PCR product for the next few cycles are shown in (h).

tify particular fragments for further analysis, such as sequencing, is available from an NIH computerized database. Almost any research laboratory has access to a facility for generating PCR primers. This approach has completely eliminated the need to actually generate and store the fragments in a centralized laboratory for distribution to interested researchers.

Approaching the Holy Grail: Large-Scale Sequencing of the Human Genome

By the end of 1995, somewhat sooner than the organizers of the Human Genome Project had originally anticipated, the molecular biology community declared itself ready to tackle the final stage of HGP: spelling out, in the language of DNA, the entire set of genetic blueprints directing the assembly and operation of a human being. The sense that it was time to begin sequencing was based on a number of considerations. The maps, both genetic and physical, were in an advanced state of readiness. In December 1995, researchers at MIT, in collaboration with French scientists, had used a PCR-based STS strategy and a variety of other techniques to produce a physical map covering ninety five percent of the human genome. STSs on this map were spaced an average of 200 kbp apart. To be sure, additional work to refine the level of precision of the maps would have to continue for another year or two, but sequencers felt the maps in hand were accurate enough to begin serious DNA sequencing on a large and coordinated scale. The initial results might only be 99.9 percent accurate—rather than the 99.99 percent originally envisioned —but the benefits of having a 99.9 percent-accurate sequence seemed to most researchers to justify an early start. Further refinements of the genetic and physical maps could continue while sequencing got underway, they argued, assuring eventual production of a 99.99 percent- accurate sequence.

A second factor—progress in sequencing the genomes of microorganisms—had proceeded extremely well. Of particular importance was the completion, in early 1996, of the sequence of the entire genome of a strain of yeast (*Saccaromyces cerevisiae*), commonly used to study molecular genetics in the laboratory. This project involved ninety laboratories in ten countries, centered mostly in Europe. Yeast cells are much closer evolutionarily to humans than the bacterial and viral genomes whose sequences had been obtained by the early 1990s. These yeast cells had sixteen chromosomes, containing approximately 6,000 genes stretched out over twelve million base pairs—about five percent of the size of the human genome. The most important aspect of this achievement for HGP was the concomitant development of technologies that will greatly increase the speed and reduce the cost of the human sequencing effort. In addition, because of the evolutionary conservation of many genes— especially those related to DNA replication and regulation of cell division —the yeast sequences will be a valuable aid in identifying many human genes encountered during human genome sequencing.

The government seemed to agree with the researchers. In April 1996, NIH announced it intended to launch a sixty-million-dollar pilot project to explore the technical feasibility of large-scale genome sequencing. The goal at present is to have the entire human genome completely sequenced by no later than the year 2005; many think it may be finished by 2003.

The way in which sequencing is proceeding in most laboratories is shown in Figure 12-3. An STS-tagged fragment associated with a particular human chromosome is digested with an appropriate restriction endonuclease into first YAC- and then cosmid-size (thirty-forty kbp) subfragments (Figure 12-3a). Each of these fragments is in turn cloned and then digested into still smaller fragments, which are cloned into plasmids. At each of these stages it will ultimately be necessary to establish the original order of each of the subfragments in the larger fragment from which it came. The way this is done is shown in detail for the final step (Figure 12-3b). Assume a given cosmid fragment is divided into only three subfragments by a particular nuclease (the restriction sites are shown by the arrows.) Each of these subfragments is sequenced, and then using that sequence information probes are made that are specific for the 3' end of each subfragment. One then takes a fresh sample of the same cosmid fragment, and digests it with a different nuclease, which generates a different set of plasmid subfragments. These are in turn cloned and sequenced, and then reacted with the probes generated at the previous step. Probe 1, which reacted with subfragment a in the first digestion, reacts with subfragment b' in the second set of subfragments. That means that subfragment b' must include the 3' end of subfragment a. Comparison of the nucleotide sequence of b' will show that it also contains the 5' end of b. That places subfragments a and b in the proper order. The same process will determine the order of b and c, and as many other subfragments as there may be in the cosmid fragment under study. Probe 3 can then be

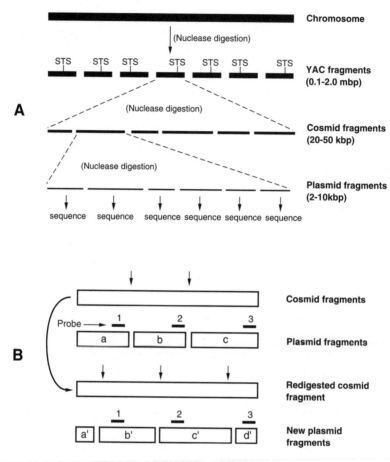

Figure 12-3. Sequencing and arranging DNA fragments.

used to define the cosmid fragment, which is a subfragment of a preceding YAC fragment. This process repeats up the ladder until the entire sequence of the starting chromosomal fragment has been determined.

How the nucleotide sequence of the final subfragments is worked out is a fairly straightforward procedure technically, and can be automated to a considerable degree. The costs of sequencing in such an enormous project are of considerable importance, and are largely related to the number of bases that can be sequenced per unit time. When HGP got underway, sequencing was extremely labor intensive, and few laboratories could sequence more than 100,000 bases per year. The cost of sequencing was in the range of five dollars per base. At that rate, it would take a hundred laboratories three hundred years to sequence the human genome, at a cost (in 1990 dollars) of fifteen billion dollars. Thus, one of HGP's major charges was to pursue the development of large-scale technologies that would increase the efficiency *and* lower the costs of DNA sequencing. It is now not unusual for a properly equipped laboratory to be able to sequence ten million bases per year, and the cost is moving toward ten cents per base.

Several strategies are underway to accelerate the gathering of useable information from sequencing of the human genome while the overall effort is still in progress. Perhaps the most interesting of these is something called *expressed sequence tags* (ESTs). The basic idea behind ESTs is that the DNA sequences of greatest immediate interest will be genes, and not the ninety-five percent or so of DNA that is noncoding. So the starting material for EST sequencing is cDNA rather than genomic DNA (cDNA, remember, is made by using the enzyme reverse transcriptase to convert mRNA into DNA). Since mRNA represents genes that are actually expressed in a cell at a given time, cDNA is essentially a pure source of gene-related (as opposed to "nonsense") DNA. Messenger RNA is harvested from a particular tissue or organ—liver, say, or brain, or bone marrow—and converted to cDNA, which is then cloned into a tissue- or organ-specific library. The resulting clones are sorted and sequenced, and the result is a catalog of genes expressed in that particular organ or tissue. Many of these will be what are called "housekeeping genes," genes that encode structural or functional proteins used in all cells simply to maintain the cell in a living state. But every tissue will reveal its own special collection of genes, used by cells in that tissue to carry out tissue-specific functions.

Already, numerous organ-specific genes have been found that were previously unknown. For example, nearly ten thousand genes have been found to be expressed at different times and under different conditions in the human brain, of which seven thousand or so are unique to the brain; over five thousand of these do not match the sequence for genes currently in the national database. Unravelling the identities and functions of these genes will almost certainly provide important new insights into how the human brain works. These cDNA clones can also be used to fish out genomic clones where the structure of the intact genes, including regulatory regions, can be studied in detail. A similar approach is being used to find genes associated with cancer. Researchers using the EST approach estimate that they may have already isolated over ninety-five percent of all human genes, although the vast majority of these have only been partially sequenced, and their function is unknown. Nevertheless, this will be a tremendously rich resource for study, and will greatly accelerate conclusion of the Human Genome Project.

As we hurtle toward the day when our voyage is concluded and the entire human genome is deciphered and laid out before us, we might well take pause and ask ourselves what we intend to do with this information. This question forms the basis of our final chapter.

13

The Ethics of
Molecular Medicine

When the implications of molecular biology for human medicine first began to dawn on those working in the field, even the molecular biologists were nervous. It was the scientists themselves, remember, who called for the Asilomar meeting in 1974, not a watchful press or wary politicians; not perennial naysayers or doomsday prophets of science. It was molecular biologists, who knew better than anyone else at the time what the stakes might be, who blew the whistle and asked for time out to sort through the implications of what they were getting themselves into. It was the scientists, and those first few physicians who understood the clinical implications of experiments still confined to bacteria and viruses, who called upon the government to take an active hand in helping regulate what they were about to do.

In the beginning, most of the concerns expressed were related to safety issues. The laboratory creation of hitherto unknown recombinant life forms—largely microbial in the beginning—created spectres of genetic monstrosities running amok in the world, causing diseases for which there might be no cure. Complex regulations were thus laid down, defining the conditions under which recombinant DNA of any kind could be used in laboratory experiments, and "biohazard containment" became the buzzphrase in molecular biology labs all over the world. A good deal of tension developed between many research universities, where nearly all of these "brave-new-world" experiments with recombinant DNA were taking place, and the surrounding communities. Both public health officials and community activists were initially suspicious of what was taking place inside these so-called "containment facilities."

But with time, concern about the immediate safety implications of research with recombinant DNA gradually subsided, first among the scientists themselves, and eventually in the public's mind as well. Special strains of *E. coli* bacteria, such as the K-12 strain, were developed for propagating cloned genes. *E. coli* had long been the favored organism for such work, largely because it is one of the most intensely studied of bacterial species, and scientists are very familiar with its inner workings. But *E. coli* lives in the human gut, and it was this fact, that spawned the concern leading to the Asilomar meeting. But K-12 is a special disabled form of *E. coli* that can survive only under closely regulated laboratory conditions. Any K-12 organism escaping from the laboratory would immediately perish.

As researchers gained experience in handling these new materials, and as NIH guidelines were revised on the basis of this experience, elaborate containment facilities were abandoned for all but the most obviously hazardous experiments. Today the vast majority of recombinant DNA research using is carried out in open laboratories on standard chemical benchtops, with no more precaution than rubber gloves and a container of bleach to throw materials into at the end of an experiment. Biologists have learned how to disable potentially harmful microbial or disease-related DNA in ways that make the DNA much safer to work with, in most cases, than the cells it came from.

While safety continues to be a primary concern of all molecular biologists, by the time the Human Genome Project was ready to get underway a number of quite different ethical questions relating specifically to molecular medicine were beginning to emerge. These concerns were not new. After some of the abortive attempts at gene therapy in the late 1970s, religious leaders had presented a united concern to the White House about such tinkering with God's work; the result was formation of a special Presidential Commission on the ethics of gene therapy. Congress established its own commission to follow developments in this new area, and to advise it on the need for appropriate regulatory legislation.

HGP itself posed a number of unique ethical problems. Knowledge is power, and even knowledge as apparently helpful as knowing the sequence of the human genome has the potential for abuse. At the very beginning of HGP, the scientists, physicians, and politicians involved in its inauguration insisted that a systematic exploration of the ethical implications of the fruits of this project be made an integral part of its operation. Thus was founded ELSI, a joint NIH/DOE Working Group on the Ethical, Legal, and Social Issues of the Human Genome Project. ELSI is supported from the operating budgets of the two parent organizations to the tune of about six million dollars per year. The members of ELSI include molecular biologists, physicians, legal experts, bioethicists, and lay persons. They are charged not only with identifying potential ethical problems and proposing possible ways of dealing with them, but also with educating the public—and other professionals such as attorneys and judges, journalists, and even "premolecular" physicians—about molecular medicine. The creation of such a group in connection with the establishment and funding of a large scientific project is unique in the annals of science, but may well be the way all such projects are carried out in the future.

Genetic Testing and Genetic Screening

One of the earliest issues to attract the attention of bioethicists, as opposed to laboratory safety officers, was the implications of molecular biology for genetic testing and genetic screening. *Genetic testing* refers to analyzing an individual for the presence or absence of specific genetic traits for which that individual is thought to be at risk. *Genetic screening* refers to analyzing individuals or populations for genetic traits without any presumption of at-risk status. By genetic "traits" we mean, ultimately, various alleles of particular genes known to be associated with disease. Molecular techniques can also be used to screen individuals or populations for infectious agents such as the AIDS virus.

Genetic testing and screening can be carried out by a variety of means. The presence of a defective gene, for example, can be detected perfectly well by measuring the presence of the corresponding defective protein, if an assay is available and samples containing the protein can readily be obtained. As DNA-based methods for detecting the presence of a particular genetic allele in a sample of DNA become available, these are generally preferred because of the ease with which such tests can be performed, and a greater degree of reliability of the results. DNA-based analyses are sometimes carried out not by testing for the gene itself, but for a closely linked marker, or RFLP. Such a test was available for Huntington's disease as early as 1983, long before the Huntington gene itself was isolated.

Direct gene sequencing as part of HGP is greatly accelerating the availability of DNA probes or PCR primers that can be used to detect genes and their variants directly. It is now possible, for example, to screen any human DNA sample for the normal CFTR gene, or for any of the subtle variants that cause the different manifestations of cystic fibrosis. The same is true for a large number of other genes associated with genetic disease. This kind of information can be of great value in many situations outside the laboratory. For example, siblings of CF and ADA-SCID patients may wish to know whether they are carriers of the corresponding defective gene. Sisters of males with X-SCID might want to know the same thing. This information, which can be obtained at any point in an individual's lifetime, can provide useful guidance for reproductive planning. Depending on the severity and treatability of the disease, and the chances of having an affected versus a healthy child, potential parents may decide to proceed with a pregnancy or select other family planning options. DNA tests on cells collected through amniocentesis can also provide information to prospective parents on the genetic status of an at-risk fetus, allowing the family and physician to plan for specialized care beginning at the moment of birth, if necessary.

Few would argue the value of genetic testing in situations of the kind just described, and in fact commercially manufactured kits are now available for routine laboratory analysis of a number of disease-associated genes. But there are potential problems associated with genetic testing that have doctors, ethicists, and the federal government genuinely concerned. The information provided by genetic testing can have profound effects on the lives of those involved, for example in the areas of health insurance and employment. It is therefore absolutely essential, first of all, that the information provided be accurate, and that both the patient and the physician (or genetic counsellor) be aware of both the implications and the limitations of this information. Medical geneticists who specialize in these questions are not always able to agree on a definitive interpretation of genetic information, and family physicians often know little more than their patients. Most major medical centers now have genetic counselling units that specialize in explaining genetic information to patients, advising them about available tests, and helping them to interpret and understand the limitations of their test results. The quality of such services will be critically important as we explore the benefits of molecular medicine. The following are a few points that every person submitting to genetic testing should demand be made as clear as possible:

Polymorphism. Genetic diseases are caused by alleles of genes that do not function correctly. In many cases there are hundreds of alleles for a given gene present in the human population. In the case of the disease-linked gene being tested for, how many alleles are known? How many of these cause disease? Are some disease-causing alleles of more concern than others? How many of these alleles will be detected in the test proposed?

Reliability. How reliable is the proposed test? Is it DNA based? If so, is the gene itself being detected, or an RFLP? (The latter always has a small inherent possibility of error.) Does the test discriminate among all of the various known disease-causing alleles? What is the history of false-positives or false-negatives of this test?

Prognosis and environment. Does having a particular allele absolutely mean disease will follow? If not, what are the probabilities? When would disease set in? To what extent do the abilities of this gene's various alleles to cause disease depend on the environment? For example, are the actions of these alleles affected by diet, smoking, drinking, or by chemicals to which you one be exposed?

Medical consequences. For diseases associated with each of the possible alleles the test can detect, what medical treatments are available? How effective are these treatments? Are the treatments experimental, or part of established medical procedure?

The implications of genetic testing and screening reach beyond individuals at risk. Consider, for example, one of the options that modern reproductive technology, when combined with molecular biology, has made available to healthy, not-at-risk parents who are carriers of potentially deadly genes. The technique of *in vitro fertilization* was developed to assist couples who have had difficulty in establishing conception through normal intercourse. In vitro fertilization involves collecting sperm and ova from the prospective parents, and mixing them together under laboratory conditions that favor fertilization (penetration of an egg by a sperm). In most cases, multiple fertilizations occur during this in vitro process, generating numerous *zygotes* (the diploid cells formed by fertilization.) The zygotes are normally monitored for several days before being reimplanted into the prospective mother's reproductive system. During this period, the zygotes undergo the initial rounds of cell division that will ultimately produce a complete human being. Zygotes that successfully begin the cell division process are referred to as *embryos*. Those embryos that appear normal under the microscope are potentially available for implantation into the prospective mother.

In those cases where one prospective parent is known to carry a potentially harmful gene, it is now possible through standard genetic screening techniques to detect the presence of this gene either in the eggs, prior to fertilization in vitro (in those cases where the mother is the sole carrier of the defective gene), or in the cells of the early embryo. During meiosis, only one of the two final meiotic cell-division products matures into a functional egg; the other meiotic daughter, which cannot be fertilized, remains physically attached to the functional ovum (Figure 13-1). This *polar body*, as it is called, can be teased away from the egg itself, and its DNA analyzed by PCR to determine its genetic status. If the mother is a carrier for, say, a defective CFTR gene, only one of the two meiotic products will carry the defective gene. Thus the genetic status of the polar body always reveals the genetic status of the functional egg: if the polar body has the defective gene, then the egg has the normal allele, and vice versa. The "molecular obstetrician" can then decide which eggs to fertilize and reimplant in the mother; the unused eggs are simply discarded.

Alternatively, fertilization can be allowed to proceed in an unselected fashion, and a number of zygotes allowed to develop into multicellular embryos. At the eight- or sixteen-cell stage of development, a single cell can be teased away from each of the embryos and analyzed by PCR. As surprising as it may seem, removal of one or two cells at this stage has absolutely no effect on the subsequent development of the embryo in vivo. After analysis of the various embryos produced, it is possible to select only those lacking the defective gene for implantation. This approach is

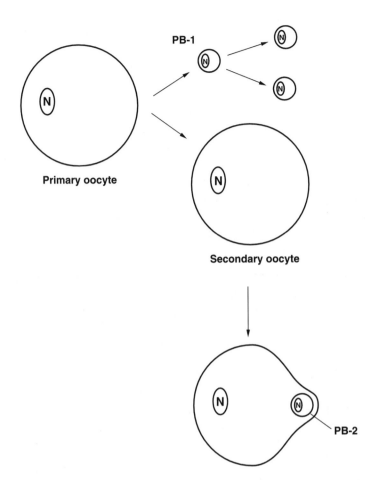

Figure 13-1. Polar body formation in human oocytes. Generation of a human egg (ovum) begins with the *primary oocyte*. All of the DNA in the nucleus (N) of the oocyte doubles, making it tetraploid (see also Figure 1-4). The cell divides, and each daughter reverts to a diploid state in terms of DNA, but the division of cellular materials is greatly unequal; the daughter that will go on to become the ovum (called a *secondary oocyte* at this stage) gets nearly all of the cellular contents. The smaller cell is known as the *first polar body* (PB-1). It divides meiotically to produce two more polar bodies; none of these plays any role in fertilization. The secondary oocyte also undergoes a meiotic cell division, producing a haploid *mature ovum*, and a haploid *second polar body* (PB-2). In humans (and most other mammals), PB-2 does not separate completely from the mature ovum. However, a skilled technician can tease it away from the ovum.

particularly useful when the father is the carrier of a harmful allele; sperm do not have an accompanying polar body for genetic prescreening.

It is obvious why this approach (which has already been used numerous times to produce disease-free infants) raises ethical concerns. While it may seem difficult to argue with sparing an unborn child the suffering that can accompany an inherited disorder such as cystic fibrosis or SCID, the techniques involved could easily be turned to other uses. In just a few more years, we will have a complete catalog of every gene in the human genome, as well as all of the variants of these genes found in the population. As the functions of these genes are sorted out, and the alterations associated with their various alleles are understood, will the "technocouple" of the future and their "gene doctor" begin to select eggs or embryos on other bases, such as physical appearance or personality traits? And what is to stop us from *adding* genes to eggs or embryos? Will future parents demand that they be allowed to scan through the catalog of the human genome, shopping for gene variants they would like to see in their children?

This is by no means a fantasy; the technology already exists. Biologists have been producing strains of genetically tailored mice, through addition of foreign genes, for over a decade. Consider too, the history of human growth hormone (HGH). The HGH protein has been produced for some years now by cloning the corresponding gene in an appropriate expression vector. Recombinant HGH was originally intended to treat children who cannot produce enough of their own, and experience a form of dwarfism as a result. But increasingly, recombinant HGH is used to treat children who are simply shorter than average and who have no underlying hormonal deficiency. What is the difference between administering a protein, and administering the gene coding for it? Why wouldn't the thinking behind nondisease use of a protein apply to the gene as well?

We should not pass too lightly over the fact that genetic manipulations carried out at the reproductive level do not affect just a single individual; they may reach far into the future. In the case of discarding embryos with known disease-causing alleles of certain genes, we are in effect purging that allele from all future members of the family involved. In the case of alleles that cause catastrophic diseases such as Huntington's chorea, it is difficult to make a case that this should not be done. But should we view diseases such as CF in the same way? What are the consequences of purging a particular form of a gene from an entire population, if we could do that? In our earlier discussion of CF, it was pointed out that the frequency of some CFTR alleles are unexplicably high in certain populations. Why is that? Could there be some unperceived advantage of the presence of these alleles, at least heterozygotically, in some populations? In the case of the variants of the β-globin gene that cause sickle cell anemia, we know that these alleles confer protection against malaria in heterozygotes (one normal and one defective globin gene), which certainly could account for their very high frequency in African peoples and their descendents. Is there some similar advantage to the ΔF-508 form of CFTR for Caucasians heterozygous at this locus? Are the circumstances in which this advantage is manifested still with us? It has, in fact, been suggested that mutant forms of CFTR may retard breast cancer development in mice and humans. Given that we can screen for this gene in at-risk individuals and provide them with reproductive counselling—and that we may well be able to correct the CFTR defect by gene therapy—ought we to rush into chasing this allele from the human species for all time?

The same considerations would apply, and even more emphatically, to the introduction of extraneous genes into human eggs or embryos. Genes introduced at these early developmental stages will show up in every cell of the resulting child, including the germ cells. This means that the added genes will be passed on to every succeeding generation. Gene products interact with each other in complex and dynamic ways that are not always well understood. It could well be that there exist allelic forms of two separate genes that by themselves do not cause disease, but when present in the same individual could cause catastrophic dysfunctions. These alleles may not normally show up in populations because they are developmentally lethal, or affect the reproductive capacity of the individual involved. What are the consequences of interfering with nature's process of keeping certain alleles apart? Considerations such as these will hopefully prevent anyone from rushing into the introduction of genes into human eggs or embryos. It is not inconceivable that we may decide that, under certain circumstances, genetic modification is acceptable or even desirable. But this is a question too large to be left to scientists alone; we must all inform ourselves of the issues, and join in the discussion.

There are also concerns about the appropriateness of genetic screening of adult populations, outside the context of reproductive planning. Some genetic diseases do not become manifest until well after birth, in some cases not until adulthood. As we have seen, cancer is not ordinarily a disease controlled by a single gene. But in a few cases, alleles have been identified that are associated with a fifty- to ninety-percent likelihood that a particular cancer will develop (some of the hereditary breast and colon cancers, for example). A gene that strongly disposes to one form of Alzheimer's disease has also been been identified. Particularly in the case of genes that predispose to specific forms of cancer that occur in middle or late life, early detection of the gene could result in much more vigilant health monitoring, leading to earlier detection and better control of the disease. But what does one do if, as in the case of Alzheimer's disease, the disease associated with an easily screenable gene is untreatable?

This dilemma has already surfaced rather dramatically in the case of Huntington's chorea. This is a disease caused by a single defective "dominant-negative" allele of an autosomal gene found on chromosome four (called IT-15) that affects brain function. Normally, IT-15 has a stretch of in-frame CAG codons that code for a poly-glutamine (poly-Gln) stretch within the IT-15 protein. In Huntington's disease this CAG stretch and the corresponding poly-Gln stretch are longer than usual; in fact, the longer the mutant stretches, the more severe and earlier-onset the disease. Apparently the extra glutamines in the protein cause it to bind to and render functionless an important cellular protein called *calmodulin*. In true dominant-negative fashion, a single mutant allele is sufficient to cause the problem.

The insertion of repeated codons in a gene, and the resulting poly-amino acid stretch in the encoded protein, occurs in other diseases as well. *Fragile X syndrome* is a severe disorder involving a gene on the X chromosome that may have a thousand or more repeats of the codon CGG, leading to the insertion of long stretches of the amino acid arginine in the middle of the Fragile X protein. Like the Huntington protein, the function of the Fragile X protein is unknown, but both disorders lead to severe disruption of mental function. Another disease with inserted codon/amino acid repeats is *myotonic dystrophy*, which contains the internal repeat CTG in the gene associated with this disease; however in this case, the repeat is contained in a portion of the gene that is not translated into protein.

Individuals born with a defective IT-15 allele are usually asymptomatic for most of their reproductive years. But once the disease sets in, it is untreatable, and the outcome is always and inevitably the same: progressive chorea (stumbling walk), dementia, and eventually death. All of the children born of a parent who succumbed to this disease are considered to be "at risk" for Huntington's disease, but on average only one-half will be carriers—and thus develop the disease themselves. The mere fact that a parent developed the disease is usually sufficient information to lead most at-risk individuals to decide not to have children. (Obviously this does not always happen, or the disease would have disappeared from the population long ago.) Should someone at risk for Huntington's disease undergo genetic testing to determine whether it is safe to have children, since the test for Huntington's disease is among those now available? Finding out that one does not carry a defective form of the gene would mean freedom from the stress of possibly developing a fatal disease. But what if the test were positive? What would one do with the knowledge that just a few years ahead lies a certain and agonizing, humiliating, painful death? The difficulty of this decision is underscored by the fact that, of the 150,000 individuals estimated to be at risk for Huntington's disease, fewer than 200 have elected to undergo the simple test that would tell them with absolute certainty whether they carry the mutated Huntington's gene. A strong consensus is developing that screening at-risk individuals or the general population for incurable or untreatable genetic diseases is inappropriate.

There is an urgent need to discuss these issues. Over 400 tests for detecting genetic diseases are currently being developed in the United States alone. Very soon, tests for the BRCA-1 gene, and tests for certain forms of Alzheimer's disease, will be on the market; other tests will surely follow. The companies producing these test kits argue that people at risk for genetic disease have an absolute right to know their genetic status. That may be, but it is not at all obvious that the public, or even most physicians, are ready to deal with the information these tests will produce, assuming it is even reliable.

Insurance, Employment, and the Right to Genetic Privacy

It is entirely conceivable that, before the middle of the next century it will be possible to analyze the DNA from just a few umbilical cord cells, and map out at birth an individual's immediate genetic past and entire genetic future—including the particular constellation of disease-associated alleles that that individual has inherited. This information could easily be stored on a tiny chip embedded in one of the plastic cards normally presented at a doctor's office or clinic. Such technology is not new; cards of this type are already in use in many health care systems, encoding important information about our general medical history. Whenever we are sick, doctors or emergency care personnel could match our symptoms against the additional genetic information stored in these chips, which could guide them to a more rapid and accurate diagnosis than is even remotely possible at present. This will almost certainly be a tremendous aid to future health care, reducing both human suffering and the costs associated with diagnosing and treating illness. But there are serious implications inherent in the very existence of this information that must be addressed if we are to profit from the many benefits such information can bring. One of the first is the issue of health insurance.

In its purest form, health insurance could be viewed as a way of evenly distributing health care costs across the population, assuring equal access to medical care at an equal cost. The overall cost of diagnosing and treating illness in any given population can be reasonably estimated based on past and anticipated health statistics, and on present and anticipated costs of medical procedures. While such estimates can be made for large populations, the ability to predict costs for individuals is more limited. Some people will go through life incurring almost no health-care costs; others will incur costs well beyond their assets plus lifetime earning power. Because no one knows for sure what his or her health status will be throughout their lifetime, and because a "pay-for-what-you-use" system would clearly bankrupt a sizeable number of individuals and families faced with catastrophic health problems, most societies have opted for some form of health-insurance system to even out the risks and costs associated with health care.

Theoretically, it should not matter whether health insurance is underwritten by the state or by private insurance companies. Both are governed by the same set of estimates for present and future health-care costs. The difference is that in a state-managed system, every citizen is guaranteed the same level of access to health care services, at the same cost. No assessment of individual risk is necessary; all participants are accepted into the plan as a right of citizenship, and all pay the same premium through taxation.

This is by no means true of private insurance systems. First of all, there is no guarantee of universal access to private health insurance; in fact, between ten and fifteen percent of the American population have no health insurance at all. Some Americans are uninsured for economic reasons: transient or chronic poverty. This is a social and political problem that of course needs to be addressed, but it is not an insurance issue per se. But some uninsured Americans have been specifically excluded from access to private health insurance protection not because of an inability to pay, but solely on the basis of information about their—or their family's—medical history and perceived medical future. Moreover, unlike state-funded insurance programs, health-care premiums may be adjusted on the basis of perceived risk to the insurer. This is standard procedure in virtually all forms of privately written insurance, whether it be for oil tankers in war-torn regions of the world, or automobile insurance in urban versus rural areas. But for health care, the result may be that even when coverage is not denied outright, the risk-adjusted cost would be so high as to effectively exclude most people on an economic basis alone. The question is whether we want to view health insurance any differently than other forms of private insurance. These and other aspects of private health insurance in America may be greatly affected by the Human Genome Project.

The most serious insurance problems arise in families that are not covered by privately underwritten group plans like those often provided as part of an employment contract. Families approaching health insurers on their own are closely examined by a prospective insurer in order to arrive at a decision about whether or not to extend policy coverage. This caution on the part of insurers is understandable; they must protect themselves from individuals who would wait until a major illness sets in, or is just over the horizon, before taking out insurance. But insurance companies in such situations also routinely exclude perfectly healthy people because they have strong family histories of hereditary diseases—sickle cell anemia or Huntington's disease, for example. In the latter case, an at-risk individual has a fifty percent likelihood of coming down with a disease that, aside from being devastating to the individual involved, will require several years of very expensive medical care. Insurance companies simply decline to write policies for such individuals; the concept of shared protection through the insurance system clearly breaks down here. Insurance companies may also exclude individuals from coverage on the basis of life-style patterns—heavy smoking or drinking in a person with a family history of heart disease, for example.

While it could be argued that the number of people dealing on their own with health-insurance companies is small, and that the future lies increasingly with large health plans where private insurers are more willing to take a distributed-risk approach, this may be begging the question. Over the coming decades, the Human Genome Project will greatly increase the number of genes known to predispose the bearer to particular diseases, and molecular medicine will make available simple, inexpensive tests to identify those genes. Any private insurance company with common sense and an eye toward reducing costs is going to want either to exclude those individuals from coverage, or to adjust their premiums to reflect the risk they represent. Heated discussions about genes such as BRCA-1 and -2 are already underway. One in three hundred women may have mutations in one or the other of these genes that can confer up to an eighty-five percent lifetime probability of breast or ovarian cancer. Companies may be willing to insure females with these gene variants while they are children, as part of a family health policy, but what private insurance company in its right mind would want to insure them once they reach adulthood, the years of greatest risk?

Yet is it really fair to allow individuals complete knowledge about their genetic makeup and predisposition to disease, and not make this same information available to a company being asked to assume the financial risks for those individuals' health care? As genetic information acquires greater predictive value, those individuals with private knowledge that they are endowed with a generally disease-free genotype could choose to pay for minimal or no health insurance, whereas those who knew they were likely to develop a serious malady during their lifetime would want maximal coverage. This would almost surely bankrupt private insurers. This is a uniquely American dilemma, for the United States alone, among the major industrialized countries of the world, relies heavily on private insurers to underwrite medical-care costs for its citizens. The present system places insurers and the insured in an adversarial situation. Insurers want as much information about potential clients as possible, so they can minimize their risk, or at least adjust premiums to reflect the risk; persons seeking insurance want to keep that information away from private insurers, for essentially the same reason.

The sense that we may have to bring about fundamental changes in the way we think about health insurance, particularly in light of the genetic revolution that HGP will force on us, was one of the first issues dealt with by the Working Group on the Ethical, Legal, and Social Issues of the Human Genome Project. In late 1995, the ELSI Working Group issued a set of guidelines on insurance issues to assist state and federal policymakers in developing legislation to ensure that "our current social, economic, and health-care policies keep pace with both the opportunities and challenges that the new genetics presents for understanding the causes of disease and developing new treatment and prevention strategies." Their major recommendations were as follows:

• Insurance providers should be prohibited from using genetic information, or even the fact that an individual may have requested such information, to deny or limit eligibility, enrollment, or continuation of health-care coverage.

• Insurance providers should be prohibited from requesting or obtaining genetic information as a requirement for considering a health-insurance application. Insurers should also be specifically enjoined from distributing any genetic information they may obtain about individual applicants to third parties without the applicant's written permission.

• Insurance providers should be prohibited from establishing differential premium rates based on genetic information, or an individual's request for genetic information. In other words, we should ensure that even in the context of private health-care underwriting, the risks and costs of genetic disorders are shared equally across all segments of society.

In an adversarial system, information is a powerful weapon—but only if it is the exclusive property of one side or the other. Genetic information as it relates to disease is going to greatly alter the relationship between insurers and the insured depending upon who controls the information. Given that insurance companies already exclude certain classes of individuals from health-care coverage on the basis of risk (or else adjust the premium to a level that excludes them economically), it is not obvious how the present system could come to grips with the challenges presented by molecular medicine without a fundamental restructuring of the entire private insurance system. Such changes are exactly what many experts are suggesting may be in order. Understandably, private insurance companies have been reluctant participants in this discussion. But they may have no choice. A dozen or so states already have legislation covering various of the points raised in the ELSI guidelines, although there is wide variation in the content and extent of individual state laws, and in the specific groups of citizens and insurers affected. But, in every case, state laws are coming down clearly on the side of the consumer on the issue of who controls genetic information.

The difficult questions that arise in connection with private insurance are part of the larger issue of "genetic privacy" raised by HGP, which will one day make possible the most detailed and intimate portrait possible of a human being. What are the implications for individuals, and their legally recognized right to privacy, of the very availability of such information? Who in society should have access to this information? What control should individuals have over this information, and under what circumstances could or should this control be contravened?

These are large questions indeed, and they are by no means esoteric. For example, employers often require a physical examination, or at least provision of information about health, as a condition of employment. The failure to meet certain health standards, or refusal to submit to the required medical tests, can be used to deny employment. How will genetic information be handled in this context? Is it any different than information about a bad back, or a possible heart or kidney problem? Employers are generally concerned about making extensive investments in training individuals who may not be able to work in peak form over the long term. If they have reason to believe someone is likely to contract a debilitating disease in the next ten years, they might not want to make such an investment. Ought they be able to include genetic information in their considerations?

Aside from issues of employment, genetic information may also play a role in providing or denying opportunities to individuals to develop their lives in certain directions. A good example was the former policy of the U.S. Air Force Academy, in force until the 1970s, of not admitting African-American cadets with sickle cell *trait*, as opposed to sickle cell *anemia*, for training as pilots and future senior officers in the Air Force. Individuals with sickle cell trait (having one normal and one dysfunctional allele for β-globin) are asymptomatic, as was known at the time, yet this genetics-based policy shut out a distinct class of citizens from a particular career opportunity. Almost certainly, other dysfunctional genetic alleles will be discovered that affect different population subgroups differently; close attention will have to be paid to the political and social — as well as the medical — implications of testing for these alleles.

222

This subject was addressed by another ELSI Working Group, which came up with proposed guidelines for a *Genetic Privacy Act.* This proposal is drafted in the language of a federal statute, and may eventually be voted into law in some form by the U.S. Congress. In the meantime, it has served as the basis for legislation in a number of states that are not content to wait for Congress to act. It is patterned after existing laws that protect access to medical information generally, but it explicitly addresses issues relating to DNA content and genetic profiles. The proposal suggests requiring authorization from any individual before a DNA sample can even be prepared from his or her tissues, for whatever purpose. The Act is aimed at protecting the individual's right to privacy, while permitting participation in genetic analysis for research and treatment purposes. It proposes that anyone collecting DNA samples from living human tissues be bound by the following rules:

- Verbal and written information about the rights of those submitting DNA samples for testing purposes must be provided *before* such samples are collected;

- DNA donors must give written authorization and consent *before* collection of specimens;

- Information about the results of any genetic tests performed on DNA samples may not be released or distributed except as authorized in writing by the donor;

- DNA samples may be used, maintained, or destroyed only as directed by the donor.

The overall intent of the Act is to ensure that the individual providing a DNA sample for genetic testing has ultimate control over the information generated from that sample, who has access to that information, and the conditions under which access may be granted.

Molecular Forensics

Forensic science, contrary to popular impressions, is not the use of medical techniques to solve crimes; it is, rather, the application of scientific and medical knowledge to legal questions. Traditionally, *forensic medicine,* a branch of forensic science, has found its widest application in determining cause of death, which is a legal matter whether or not a crime is involved or even suspected. It is thus a specialization of pathology, and uses the pathologist's skills at autopsy, in the microscopic examination of tissues, and in the toxicological analysis of tissues and fluids. Forensic pathologists may also be called upon to render opinions about paternity, or the identification of human remains, as an aid to legal inquiries.

More recently, forensic scientists find themselves increasingly called upon to render opinions about the ability of DNA samples to establish the identity of individuals in legal matters. Quite often the legal matter does involve a crime, and the object is to examine the DNA content of a blood or tissue sample found at a crime scene, and calculate the probability that a particular individual suspected of the crime was likely to have left those samples. But DNA is also used to identify victims of accidents or military action, and may be used in paternity matters as well.

Obviously, if we had a complete genomic sequence recorded for every member of society, these questions would hardly require scientific experts to testify in court; a computer could resolve the question in a matter of seconds. But we do not have this information at present, and we may never have it (for social and political as well as scientific reasons) and so we will have to make do with the advice of geneticists and molecular biologists for the foreseeable future. As we shall see, we will be very dependent on the advice of biostatisticians as well.

The basic strategy behind DNA testing for identification purposes is fairly straightforward. The human genome is a remarkable mixture of consistency and variation between individuals. The nucleotide sequences of functional genes tend to be highly conserved among individuals, yet they clearly do have differences—for example the minor allelic variations that cause disease. It is these polymorphisms that account for the phenotypic differences among human beings; without them, essentially, we would all be identical twins. The sequence of that portion of the genome not coding for functional genes is much less rigorously conserved: it is much more polymorphic. It has been estimated that humans differ from one another in at least one nucleotide per thousand, on average. In one sense that is a tribute to the remarkable fidelity of DNA reproduction from generation to generation; on the other hand, it means that there are several million base pairs of difference between most unrelated individuals. By comparing two DNA samples for the exact array of alleles present for a selected number of polymorphic loci—whether genes or RFLPs— we can make reasonable estimates about the genetic relatedness of the two samples. The idea of using polymorphism in this way is not new; ABO and Rh blood groups are based on polymorphisms, as are the slightly different forms of the same blood protein found in different individuals. What is new is lowering the level of analysis to the DNA itself, where all of these polymorphisms originate.

The system most commonly used at present for comparing human DNA samples is based on the STRs (short tandem repeats) of which it has been estimated that the human genome may contain as many as half a million. The function of these blocks of nucleotide repeats is largely unknown. STRs based on motifs of seven to fifteen nucleotides are most often associated with the centromeric regions of chromosomes (see Figure 7-1), and may simply play a structural role in chromosomal organization. The STRs most commonly used for forensic analysis, however, are end-to-end repeats (twenty-five to one hundred copies) of shorter (three to five bp) nucleotide sequences. These sequences are scattered widely throughout the genome. Some may occur as part of the coding portion of functional genes—the trinucleotide repeat CAG that occurs in the Huntington gene and encodes polyglutamine, for example—but most are found in the middle of so-called "nonsense" DNA, which has no known function.

Most of these STRs have easily identifiable "alleles" in the human population. These alleles are based not on minute differences in the STR nucleotide sequence, as was the case for RFLPs (see Figure 12-1), but rather on the *number of repeats* in the basic nucleotide repeat unit defining the STR. For that reason, STRs are also referred to by the name "variable number of tandem repeats," or VNTR. STRs render the same kind of information about individuals and heredity as would an analysis of real genes, or of RFLPs. STRs are genetically stable; that is, they are passed to offspring with exactly the same number of repeats present in the parent. Moreover, STR alleles are distributed slightly differently in different human racial subgroups, mimicking in yet another way the behavior of classical gene alleles.

The application of PCR technology to STR analysis has revolutionized the ability of forensic technicians to identify the origin of extremely minute samples of hair, skin, semen, and other human tissues. Analyses can be (and have been) carried out on a single hair root, the lip cells left on a cigarette tip, or the saliva on the back of a postage stamp. Up until a few years ago, identification of individuals from their DNA was done by Southern analysis of RFLPs (see pp. 192–196). These were the basis for the DNA information presented in the O. J. Simpson trial, for example. But RFLP analysis is slow, requires relatively large DNA samples, and is very sensitive to damage that may have been done to the sample. However, PCR analysis of STRs requires a hundred to a thousand times less DNA, can be performed quickly and simply with relatively few errors, and is less sensitive to degradation of the sample. This method of analysis will certainly be preferred for forensic matters in the future.

The way STR analysis works is shown in Figure 13-2. Let us consider two STR loci: HumCD4 and HumARA. HumCD4 is found on chromosome twelve, and HumARA is found on chromosome thirteen. These STRs, and the DNA that surrounds them in the genome, have been

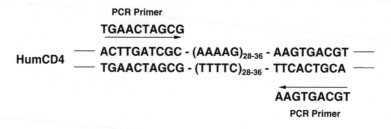

PCR Primer

TGAACTAGCG

HumCD4 —— ACTTGATCGC - (AAAAG)$_{28\text{-}36}$ - AAGTGACGT ——
—— TGAACTAGCG - (TTTTC)$_{28\text{-}36}$ - TTCACTGCA ——

AAGTGACGT

PCR Primer

HumCD4			
std	A	B	C
(28) —			
(29) —			
(30) —		—	
(31) —	—		
(32) —		—	
(33) —			—
(34) —			
(35) —	—		
(36) —			

HumARA			
std	A	B	C
(86) —	—		
(88) —			
(90) —		—	
(92) —	—		—
(94) —			
(96) —			—
(98) —			
(100) —		—	
(102) —			
(104) —			

Figure 13-2. The use of short tandem repeats (STRs) in comparing human DNA samples.

226

sequenced. The basic HumCD4 repeat unit is $(AAAAG)_n$, where n can range between twenty-eight and thirty-six in different alleles. The AGC nucleotide motif defining the HumARA STR can be repeated 85 to 105 times. Using PCR primers specific for the DNA sequences known to lie on either side of defined STR sites, the DNA from an individual can be analyzed by running the PCR products of that individual's DNA on a standard electrophoresis gel, and comparing the resulting bands with known size standards. The PCR products will reflect very precisely the number of repeats associated with a given DNA sample, allowing assignment of specific allele designations.

In the example shown in Figure 13-2, individuals A and B are both heterozygous at both loci. One of A's chromosomes has HumCD4 repeated thirty-one times, and the other chromosome has thirty-five repeats. When A's DNA is collected, both chromosomes (one maternally, and the other paternally, inherited) are of course present, and in A's case two physically distinguishable versions of the HumCD4 locus are detectable. We would say that individual A is heterozygous at the HumCD4 locus, just as A might be heterozygous for the CF or SCID gene locus. Individual B is also heterozygous at these two loci, and all of B's alleles at these loci are different from those of A. Individual C is homozygous at the HumCD4 locus, but heterozygous at HumARA. One of C's alleles at HumARA is the same as one of A's alleles at this locus.

The number of different alleles at the STR loci used for DNA typing is most often between ten and twenty, which gives a greater than seventy percent likelihood on average that an individual will be heterozygous at these loci. This is important because it bears on the likelihood of two DNA samples being identical. Let us assume that two samples of DNA are compared by analysing a panel of five different STR loci, which is not uncommon. One of these samples, X, was taken from a crime scene and is presumed to have been left by the person committing the crime (e.g., foreign skin found under the fingernails of the victim). The other sample, Y, is collected from a suspect in the crime. For sake of simplicity, let us assume that both samples show heterozygosity at all five loci. If even one of the alleles at any of the five loci tested is different, the matter is immediately resolved, without discussion. The samples could not have come from the same individual, and Y did not leave the samples collected at the crime scene. DNA evidence is very clear in this respect, and a number of individuals charged with a crime, and quite a few who had already been convicted of a crime and sent to prison (thirty-six who had been on death row, through 1996), have been exonerated by DNA analyses.

But now suppose that all ten alleles analyzed were absolutely identical in the two samples. What is the probability that samples X and Y came from the same individual? Or as a statistician would rather put it, what is the probability that the samples could have come from two *different* individuals? That is the question on which virtually all legal matters involving DNA evidence turn. It is approached in the following way. For each of the loci involved, the likelihood that a particular genotype (i.e., a particular combination of alleles) will show up in the same person is known, because it has been studied in large numbers of people, and the information stored in a DNA typing database. Let us say that for Y, the suspect, the probability of finding his combination of alleles at locus one is one in twenty. For loci two through five, the probabilities are one in twelve, fifteen, twenty-two, and eighteen, respectively. Then the overall probability that someone *else*—someone other than Y—would have exactly the same set of alleles as those found in the crime scene sample would appear to be one-in-twenty x one-in-twelve x one-in-fifteen x one-in-twenty-two x one-in-eighteen, or 1,425,600. So the probability is not zero, but it is extremely low. By increasing the number of loci tested to seven, instead of five, the probability that someone other than Y left the sample at the crime scene would begin to approach the number of people living in the United States.

But some have claimed that the analysis may not be quite so straightforward. For one thing, STR alleles are distributed differently in different racial subgroups. It is thus possible that someone in a racial subgroup different from Y's could have a higher likelihood of having the identical set of alleles for the loci tested. The defense would thus want to present the calculation for the racial subgroup with the highest probability (assuming it was a subgroup different from Y's; otherwise we can count on the prosecution making this point.) In fact when large numbers of loci (five or more) are tested such differences tend to disappear, but it is certainly important to ask the computer to do all of the relevant calculations.

It has also been argued that it may not be appropriate to calculate the probability of matching alleles at several loci by simply multiplying the probabilities at each locus. Doing so is appropriate if the loci are truly independent of one another, but do we know that the STR loci being tested do behave in a truly independent fashion? If each locus in a test panel is located on a different chromosome, the loci will in fact behave largely independent of one another. It has also been argued that even genes on different chromosomes can influence one another's selection. For example, most proteins in a cell interact with at least one other protein. Certain variants of proteins produced by specific alleles of the genes involved may work together better than other variants encoded by other alleles, giving a survival or reproductive advantage to bearers of certain allelic combinations. This is a form of functional, as opposed to physical, gene linkage. Thus one advantage of typing STRs as opposed to real genes is that most STRs do not encode anything (those that do can be avoided), and particular STR combinations will not have been acted on by natural selection. If they are unlinked physically, then they should operate independently, simplifying the accompanying statistical calculations.

In the end, it is impossible to say that having a particular allele at one locus absolutely will not influence which allele is found at a second locus, but so far no such interactions involving STRs have been found. As the technology for analyzing STRs by PCR continues to improve, it will become possible to establish identities or nonidentities of DNA samples with statistically overwhelming precision. When we can say that fewer than one person in five billion could have had a given panel of allelic variants and still be different than the accused, statistical arguments in a world of five billion people cease to be meaningful. But we must somehow educate judges, attorneys, and citizens who serve as jurors about the subtleties of DNA evidence and its analysis. And for the present we remain haunted by the fact that the absolutely unambiguous DNA test —a negative match—can grant someone freedom; the result that may lock someone up for life—or possibly lead to his or her death—will be based on manipulation of numbers for the foreseeable future. Until we can truly render statistical arguments meaningless, we would do well to err on the side of caution.

The use of DNA typing in forensic matters also intersects with concerns about genetic privacy, especially since something called the DNA Identification Act became law in late 1994 as part of a larger federal crime bill. The Federal Bureau of Investigation now maintains a nationwide DNA identification file named CODIS (combined DNA index system). The basic idea is that whenever state or local authorities type a criminal's DNA, the information about that individuals's DNA will be stored in a central file, where it will be available to law enforcement agencies in other states and, with permission of the FBI, to international agencies as well. At the present time, arrival of information to CODIS from agencies around the country has been slow, except from California and Virginia where such programs were underway before 1994. However, forty-one states have passed legislation requiring convicted offenders to submit DNA samples for the database. The reasons for slow growth at this point have to do only with development of adequate technologies in the contributing laboratories, not with any concern about the appropriateness of collecting and pooling such information per se. Indeed, from a purely law enforcement point of view, the ability to track and identify known criminals through the minutest traces of biological materials has great appeal, and will certainly go a long way to facilitate catching repeat offenders. CODIS has already been used to identify perpetraters of crimes in cases where there were simply no suspects until tissue samples left at the scene were analyzed and matched with CODIS files. Even when a specific individual cannot be personally identified, the same DNA left at two different crime scenes can tell investigators that the same individual was almost certainly involved in both crimes.

The DNA Identification Act provides funds to bring crime labs around the country up to speed in DNA technology, and the advent of PCR/STR strategies will make this money go a great deal further than originally expected. (Virtually all of the DNA typing by crime labs through 1995 or so was based on RFLP analysis; these samples will almost certainly have to be reanalyzed by PCR/STR for future use.) In 1996, the federal government targeted an additional forty million dollars to upgrade CODIS and make it easier to use. Therefore, we can expect to see rapid growth in CODIS in the next few years. But the very existence of such a centralized file should raises a number of legitimate concerns. Who exactly will this information be collected from? What exactly will be done with it? How long will it be kept? What are the limitations on its use and its distribution to third parties? Is such an information bank any different from the centralized fingerprint file maintained by the FBI? What happens to genetic information about individuals later released for lack of evidence, or who are declared innocent by a jury?

If there is a common thread running through the discussions about the ethics of molecular medicine, and particularly the issues raised by the Human Genome Project, it is this: We must never allow molecular genetics to be used by any one group—whether defined economically, socially, racially, or by any other criterion — to enhance or even consolidate its position in the body politic. Nor must we ever allow individuals defined by molecular genetics as somehow different from the "norm," on whatever basis, to be put at risk for selective and potentially prejudicial treatment. To the extent that information about genetic constitution is ever used to identify, isolate, or diminish any one segment of society to the advantage of another, all of the potential benefits of this astounding revolution in human medicine could be lost in a political backlash the likes of which we may never have seen. These benefits are too important to all of us to let this happen. Every segment of society — doctors, scientists, legal experts, ethicists, and most importantly, common citizens — must make themselves aware of the underlying problems and possible solutions, and join in the debate that will decide these issues as we enter the twenty-first century.

Further Reading

1. In the Beginning

Mendel, G. Experiments in Plant Hybridization. In: *Mendel Centenary: Genetics, Development and Evolution* (R. Nardone, ed.). The Catholic University of America Press, Washington D.C., 1968.

Moore, J. A. *Science As a Way of Knowing: The Foundations of Modern Biology.* Harvard University Press, Cambridge, MA, 1993.

Olby, R. *Origins of Mendelism.* University of Chicago Press, Chicago, 1985.

2. Cystic Fibrosis

Goodfellow, P. (ed.). *Cystic Fibrosis.* Oxford University Press, Oxford and New York, 1989.

Welsh, M., and A. Smith. Cystic Fibrosis. *Scientific American* 273:52 (1996).

3. DNA and the Language of Genes

Avery, O. T., C. M. MacLeod, and M. McCarty. Studies on the Nature of the Substance Inducing Transformation of Pneumococcal Types. *Journal of Experimental Medicine* 79:137 (1944).

Hershey, A. D., and M. Chase. Independent Functions of Viral Protein and Nucleic Acid in Growth of Bacteriophage. *Journal of General Physiology* 36:39 (1952).

Judson, H. F. *The Eighth Day of Creation.* Simon & Schuster, New York, 1979.

Schrödinger, E. *What Is Life?* Cambridge University Press, Cambridge and New York, 1944.

Watson, J., and F. Crick. Genetic Implications of the Structure of Deoxyribonucleic Acid. *Nature* 171:964 (1953).

Ibid. Molecular Structure of Nucleic Acids: A Structure for Deoxynucleic Acids. *Nature* 171:738 (1953).

4. Severe Combined Immunodeficiency Disease

Clark, W. R. *At War Within; The Double-Edged Sword of the Immune System,* Oxford University Press, Oxford and New York, 1995.

Stiehm, R. (ed.). *Immune Disorders in Infants and Children,* 4th edition. W. B. Saunders, Philadelphia, 1996.

5. The Isolation, Cloning, and Transfer of Human Genes

Lodish, H., et al. *Molecular Cell Biology, 3rd edition.* W. H. Freeman & Co., New York, 1995.

Nathans, D., and H. Smith. Restriction Endonucleases in the Analysis and Restructuring of DNA

Molecules. *Annual Reviews of Biochemistry* 44:273 (1975).

Morgan, T. H. *The Theory of the Gene.* Yale University Press, New Haven, 1926.

Smith, A. Viral Vectors in Gene Therapy. *Annual Reviews of Microbiology* 49:807 (1995).

Southern, E. Detection of Specific Sequences Among DNA Fragments Separated by Gele Electrophoresis. *Journal of Molecular Biology* 98:503 (1975).

Watson, J. D., *The Double Helix.* Atheneum Press, New York, 1968.

Watson, J. D., N. Hopkins, J. Roberts, J. Steitz, and A. Weiner. *Molecular Biology of the Gene,.* 4th Edition. Benjamin/Cummings, Menlo Park, 1990.

6. The Journey Begins: The Clinical Trials for ADA-SCID

Blaese, R. M., K. W. Culver, et al.T Lymphocyte-Directed Gene Therapy for ADA-SCID: Initial Trial Results after Four Years. *Science* 270:475 (1995).

Bordignon, C. et al. Gene Therapy in Peripheral Blood Lymphocytes and Bone Marrow for ADA-Deficient Patients. *Science* 270:470 (1995).

Kohn, D. B. et al. Engraftment of Gene-Modified Umbilical Cord Blood Cells in Neonates with Adenosine Deaminase Deficiency. *Nature Medicine* 1:1017 (1995).

Leonard, W., M. Noguchi, S. Russell and O. McBride. The Molecular Basis of X-linked Severe Combined Immunodeficiency: The Role of the Interleukin-2 Receptor γ-chain. *Immunological Reviews* 138:61 (1994).

Lyon, J., and P. Gorner. *Altered Fates: Gene Therapy and the Retooling of Human Life.* W. W. Norton, New York, 1995.

Orkin, S., P. Daddona, D. Shewach, A. Markham, G. Bruns, S. Goff, and W. Kelley. Molecular Cloning of the Adenosine Deaminase Gene. *Journal of Biological Chemistry* 258:12753 (1983).

Qazilbash, M. et al. Retroviral Vector for Gene Therapy of X-linked Severe Combined Immunodeficiency Syndrome. *Journal of Hematotherapy* 4:91 (1995).

7. The Clinical Trials for Cystic Fibrosis

Caplen, N., et al. Liposome-Mediated CFTR Gene Transfer to the Nasal Epithelium of Patients with Cystic Fibrosis. *Nature Medicine* 1:39 (1995).

Crystal, R. G. Administration of an Adenovirus Containing the Human CFTR cDNA to the Respiratory Tract of Individuals with Cystic Fibrosis. *Nature Genetics* 8:42 (1994).

Knowles, M., et al. A Controlled Study of Adenoviral Vector-Mediated Gene Transfer in the Nasal Epithelium of Patients with Cystic Fibrosis. *New England Journal of Medicine* 333:823 (1995).

Rommens, J., et al. Identification of the Cystic Fibrosis Gene: Chromosome Walking and Jumping. *Science* 245:1059 (1989).

Tsui, L.-C.. The Cystic Fibrosis Transmembrane Conductance Regulator Gene. *American Journal of Respiratory and Critical Care Medicine* 151:S47 (1995).

8. Gene Therapy for Monogenic Disorders

Bauters, C. Gene Therapy for Cardiovascular Disease. *European Heart Journal* 16:1166 (1995).

Emerman, M. From Curse to Cure: HIV for Gene Therapy? *Nature Biotechnology* 14:943 (1995).

Fairbairn, L., et al. Long-Term in vitro Correction of α-L-iduronidase Deficiency (Hurler syndrome) in Human Bone Marrow. *Proceedings National Academy of Sciences* 93:2025 (1996).

Felgner, P. Improvements in Cationic Liposomes for in vivo Gene Transfer. *Human Gene Therapy* 7:1791 (1996).

Friedmann, T. Human Gene Therapy—An Immature Genie, but Certainly Out of the Bottle. *Nature Medicine* 2:144 (1996).

Grossman, M., et al. Successful ex vivo Gene Therapy Directed to the Liver in a Patient with Familial Hypercholesterolemia. *Nature Genetics* 6:335 (1994).

Hodgson, C., and F. Solaiman. Virosomes: Cationic Liposomes Enhance Retroviral Transduction. *Nature Biotechnology* 14:339 (1996).

Isner, J., et al. Clinical Evidence of Angiogenesis after Arterial Gene Transfer of phVEGF in a Patient with Ischemic Limb. *The Lancet* 348:370 (1996).

Smith, R. et al. Pharmacokinetics and Tolerability of Venticularly Administered Superoxide Dismutase in Monkeys and Preliminary Clinical Observations in Familial ALS. *Journal of Neurological Sciences* 129 (suppl. 13):8 (1995).

Van Beusechem, V. and D. Valerio. Gene Transfer into Hematopoietic Stem Cells of Nonhuman Primates. *Human Gene Therapy* 7:1649 (1996).

Zhang, W. Antisense Oncogene and Tumor Suppressor Gene Therapy of Cancer. *J. Molecular Medicine* 74:191 (1996)

9. Gene Therapy for Cancer

Clark, W. R. *At War Within: The Double-Edged Sword of the Immune System.* New York: Oxford University Press, 1995.

Clayman, G. Gene Therapy for Head and Neck Cancer. *Head and Neck* 17:535 (1995).

Folkman, J. Fighting Cancer by Attacking its Blood Supply. *Scientific American*, September 1996, p. 150.

Freeman, S., et al. In Situ Use of Suicide Genes for Cancer Treatment. *Seminars in Oncology* 23:31 (1996).

Herrmann, F. Cancer Gene Therapy: Principles, Problems and Perspectives. *Journal of Molecular Medicine* 73:157 (1995).

Holt, J., et al. Gene Therapy for the Treatment of Metastatic Breast Cancer by in vivo Transduction with Breast-Targeted Retroviral Vector Expressing c-FOS Antisense. *Human Gene Therapy* 7:1367 (1996).

Maron, A., et al. Gene Therapy of Rat Glioma Using Adenovirus-Mediated Transfer of the Herpes Simplex Virus Thymidine Kinase Gene: Longterm Followup by Magnetic Resonance Imaging. *Gene Therapy* 3:315 (1996).

Miki, Y., et al. A Strong Candidate for the Breast and Ovarian Cancer Susceptibility Gene BRCA1. *Science* 266:66 (1994).

Roth, J. Gene Replacement Strategies for Cancer. *Israel Journal of Medicine* 32:89 (1996).

Roth, J., et al. Retrovirus-Mediated Wild-Type p53 Gene Transfer to Tumors of Patients with Lung Cancer. *Nature Medicine* 2:985 (1996).

Tong, X., et al. In vivo Gene Therapy of Ovarian Cancer by Adenovirus-Mediated Thymidine Kinase Gene Transduction and Gancyclovir Administration. *Gynecologic Oncology* 61:175 (1996).

Wooster, R., et al. Identification of the Breast Cancer Susceptibility Gene BRCA2. *Nature* 378:789 (1995).

Zhang, W. Antisense Oncogene and Tumor Suppressor Gene Therapy of Cancer. *Journal of Molecular Medicine* 4:191. (1996).

10. Molecular Medicine and AIDS

Caruso, M., and D. Klatzmann. Selective Killing of CD4[+] Cells Harboring an HIV-Inducible Suicide Gene Prevents Viral Spread in an Infected Cell Population. *Proceedings National Academy of Sciences (USA)* 89:182 (1992).

Marasco, W. et al. Design, Intracellular Expression and Activity of a Human Anti-HIV-1 gp120 Single-Chain Antibody. *Proceedings National Academy of Sciences* 90:7889 (1993).

Morgan, R. Gene Therapy for AIDS Using Retroviral Mediated Gene Transfer to Deliver HIV Antisense TAR and Transdominant Rev Protein Genes to Syngeneic Lymphocytes in HIV-Infected Identical Twins. *Human Gene Therapy* 7:1281 (1996).

Moutouh, L., J. Corbeil, and D. Richman. Recombination Leads to the Rapid Emergence of HIV-1 Dually Resistant Mutants Under Selective Drug Pressure. *Proceedings National Academy of Sciences* 93:6106 (1996).

Ragheb, J., et al. Analysis of Trans-Dominant Mutants of the HIV Type 1 Rev Protein for their Ability to Inhibit Rev Function, HIV Type 1 Replication, and Their Use as Anti-HIV Gene Therapeutics. *AIDS Research and Retroviruses* 11:1343 (1995).

Woffendin, C., et al. Expression of a Protective Gene Prolongs Survival of T cells in HIV-Infected

Patients. *Proceedings National Academy of Sciences* 93:2889 (1996).

11. Naked DNA

Bourne, N., et al. DNA Immunization Against Experimental Genital Herpes Simplex Virus Infection. *Journal of Infectious Diseases* 173:800 (1996).

Davis, H., et al. DNA-Mediated Immunization in Mice Induces a Potent MHC Class I-Restricted Cytotoxic T Lymphocyte Response to the Hepatitis B Envelope Protein. *Human Gene Therapy* 6:1447 (1995).

Davis, H., et al. DNA Vaccine for Hepatitis B: Evidence for Immunogenicity in Chimpanzees and Comparison with Other Vaccines. *Proceedings National Academy of Sciences* 93:7213 (1996).

Tascon, R., et al. Vaccination Against Tuberculosis by DNA Injection. *Nature Medicine* 2:888 (1996).

Whalen, R. G. DNA Vaccines for Emerging Infectious Diseases: What If? *Emerging Infectious Diseases* 2:168 (1996).

12. The Human Genome Project

Bishop, J., and M. Waldholz. Genome. Touchstone/Simon & Schuster, New York, 1990.

Botstein, D. et al. Construction of a Genetic Linkage Map in Man Using Restriction Fragment Length Polymorphism. *American Journal of Human Genetics* 32:314 (1980).

Gibbs, R. A. Pressing Ahead with Human Genome Sequencing. *Nature Genetics* 11:121 (1995).

Hudson, T. J., et al. An STS-based Map of the Human Genome. *Science* 270:1945 (1995).

Kevles, D., and L. Hood (eds.). *The Code of Codes*. Harvard University Press, Cambridge, MA, 1992.

National Research Council. *Mapping and Sequencing the Human Genome*. National Academy Press, Washington D.C., 1988.

13. The Ethics of Molecular Medicine

Abraham, E., et al. Cystic Fibrosis Hetero- and Homozygosity is Associated with Inhibition of Breast Cancer Growth. *Nature Medicine* 2:593 (1996).

Bao, J. et al. Expansion of Polyglutamine Repeat in Huntingtin Leads to Abnormal Protein Interactions Involving Calmodulin. *Proceedings of the National Academy of Sciences* 93:5037 (1996).

Fregeau, C., and R. Fourney. DNA Typing with Fluorescently Tagged Short Tandem Repeats: a Sensitive and Accurate Approach to Human Identification. *BioTechniques* 15:100 (1993).

Hudson, K. Genetic Discrimination and Health Insurance: An Urgent Need for Reform. *Science* 270:391 (1995).

Kitcher, P. *The Lives to Come*. Simon & Schuster, New York, 1996.

Lee, H., et al. DNA Typing in Forensic Science. Theory and Background. *Amer. Journal of Forensic Medicine and Pathology* 15:269 (1994).

McEwen, J. E. Forensic DNA Data Banking by State Crime Laboratories. *American Journal of Human Genetics* 56:1487 (1994).

Micka, K. et al. Validation of Multiplex Polymorphic STR Amplification Sets Developed for Personal Identification Applications. *Journal of Forensic Sciences* 41:582 (1996).

Glossary

ADA Adenosine deaminase

Allele Normal or mutated variant of a gene present in a given species

Amino acid Small organic molecule that is the building block for proteins

Angiogenesis Generation of blood vessels

Apoptosis The sequence of events involved in programmed cell death

Autosome Any of the chromosomes except the sex chromosomes

AZT Azidothymidine, a drug used to treat HIV infection

BAC Bacterial artificial chromosome, used for cloning DNA

Bacteriophage Virus that reproduces itself in a bacterium

Base Alternate term for nucleotide

Base pair A unit of size for measuring DNA, equivalent to the length of one pair of complementary nucleotides on opposing DNA strands

Carrier In heredity, an individual carrying one copy of an altered gene

cDNA Complementary DNA, made by reverse transcription of RNA

CFTR Cystic fibrosis transport regulator; the gene mutated in cystic fibrosis

Chromatin The DNA and protein comprising a chromosome

Chromosome A structure present in the nucleus, composed of DNA and protein, containing the genes

Clone Cells derived from a single cellular precursor; also used to mean exogenous DNA replicated in a clone of cells

Codon A sequence of three nucleotides specifying an amino acid

CODIS Combined DNA Index System; DNA file maintained by the FBI

Complementary DNA DNA made by copying mRNA with reverse transcriptase

Cord blood Blood obtained from the umbilical cord at birth

Cosmid A large cloning vector made from a bacteriophage

Crossing over The exchange of segments of DNA between two homologous chromosomes

Cytokine A hormone-like molecule used by cells to communicate with one another

ddC Dideoxycytosine, a drug used to combat HIV infection

ddI Dideoxyinosine, a drug used to combat HIV infection

Diploid Having the normal amount of DNA per cell, ie two copies of each chromosome

DNA polymerase The enzyme responsible for DNA replication

Downstream In a gene, the 3' direction of the nucleotide sequence

dscDNA Double-stranded cDNA

ELSI Joint NIH-DOE Working Group on the Ethical, Legal, and Social Issues associated with the Human Genome Project

Episome DNA that is not incorporated into the genome, but is replicated together with the genome
EST Expressed sequence tag
Exon The coding portion of a gene
Ex vivo Outside the body

Frameshift mutation An alteration in the nucleotide sequence of a gene that causes the reading frame to be altered

Gemmules The physically discrete elements proposed by Darwin to be responsible for heredity
GenBank Federal repository for DNA sequences, available to all researchers
Gene Segment of DNA encoding a protein or functional RNA molecule
Gene linkage The presence of two genes on the same chromosome
Genome The entire collection of genes possessed by an individual
Genotype The particular collection of alleles for each gene in an individual
Germ cell Cell responsible for transmitting DNA to the next generation

Haploid Having one-half the normal amount of DNA per cell, e.g. one set of chromosomes
Heterozygote Having two different alleles of a given gene
Homozygote Having the same two alleles of a given gene
Housekeeping gene Gene actively expressed in all cells of the body
Hstk *Herpes simplex* thymidine kinase
Hybridization Association of two strands of nucleic acid according to the A/T, G/C rule

Idiopathic disease Disease arising from within the organism
Interleukin Cytokine used by cells of the immune system
Insertional mutagenesis Mutations caused by exogenous DNA inserting into a genome
Intron Noncoding regions of DNA separating the exons of a gene
In vivo Inside a living body
IRB Institutional review board; an in-house committee that reviews research proposals for compliance with federal regulations before submission to a federal agency

Kilobase pairs One thousand base pairs

Liposome Small fat body used to deliver DNA or other drugs to cells

Meconium The mucoid substance present in the intestines of a newborn; normally eliminated in the first defecation
Meiosis Cell division in which the DNA content is first reduced by half
mRNA Messenger RNA, a copy of a DNA gene, used by the cell to manufacture a protein
Mitochonrion The organelle responsible for energy production in a cell
Mitosis Cell division
MoMLV Moloney murine leukemia virus
Mutagen Any substance causing a change in the nucleotide sequence of a gene
Mutation An alteration in the nucleotide sequence of a gene; may or may not result in an altered phenotype

NIH National Institutes of Health
Nonsense DNA DNA sequences, such as introns, that have no coding function
Nuclein The original name given to DNA
Nucleotide Small organic molecules forming the building blocks of DNA and RNA

Oncogene A gene involved in cellular signal transduction which, when mutated, disposes toward cancer
Open reading frame Promoter region and/or start codons indicating presence of a gene

238

Opportunistic infection An infection caused by an agent already present in the body, normally kept under control by the immune system

Organelle The internal structures of a cell responsible for carrying out the functions of that cell

ORF Open reading frame

Packaging cell Cell containing DNA sequences missing from a virus, used to produce completed copies of the virus

Pathogenic Causing disease

PCR Polymerase chain reaction, a technique for amplifying small stretches of DNA

PEG-ADA Polyethylene glycol chemically coupled to ADA

Peptide A small protein or fragment thereof

Phage A bacteriophage

Phenotype The observable physical and chemical properties of an individual, as determined by that individual's genotype

Plasmid A stable episome in bacteria

Point mutation Change in a single nucleotide in the sequence of a gene

Probe Small piece of DNA used to identify by hybridization the corresponding sequence in a DNA sample

Promoter Region immediately upstream of a gene that regulate its expression in a cell

Provirus cDNA copy of a retroviral RNA genome

RAC Recombinant DNA Advisory Committee; NIH committee charged with reviewing research proposals using recombinant DNA

Recombinant DNA A hybrid molecule using DNA from two different sources

Recombinant protein A protein derived from recombinant DNA

Restriction endonuclease An enzyme that cuts DNA at specific nucleotide motifs

Restriction fragment DNA fragment resulting from digestion of DNA with a restriction endonuclease

Retrovirus RNA virus that reverse transcribes its RNA into a cDNA provirus, which is then incorporated into the host genome

RFLP Restriction fragment length polymorphism

Ribosome Organelle where proteins are made

RNA polymerase The enzyme that copies DNA into RNA

Southern analysis Technique for separating and identifying DNA restriction fragments by size

STR Short tandem repeat

STS Sequence-tagged site

Tetraploid Having double the normal (diploid) amount of DNA in a cell

TNF Tumor necrosis factor, an interleukin that kills tumor cells

Transcription Copying of DNA into RNA using DNA polymerase

Transfection Transfer of functional DNA into a cell

Transgene Exogenous gene introduced into the genome of another organism

Translation Conversion of a messenger RNA to the corresponding protein

Tumor suppressor gene Gene that blocks unscheduled cell division

Upstream In a gene, the 5' direction of the nucleotide sequence

Vector A virus or other agent used to deliver DNA to a cell

VNTR Variable number of tandem repeats

YAC Yeast artificial chromosome

Zygote The diploid cell formed as the result of union of a haploid sperm and ovum

Index